Mental Health, Psychiatry and the Arts

Mental Health, Psychiatry and the Arts

A TEACHING HANDBOOK

Edited by

VICTORIA TISCHLER

CPsychol, BSW, MSocSc, PhD, PGCHE
University of Nottingham
Division of Psychiatry-Behavioural Sciences
Queen's Medical Centre
Nottingham

Forewords by

DINESH BHUGRA

Professor of Mental Health & Cultural Diversity
Institute of Psychiatry, King's College London
President, Royal College of Psychiatrists

and

ALLAN D PETERKIN

Associate Professor of Psychiatry and Family Medicine
University of Toronto

Radcliffe Publishing
Oxford • New York

Radcliffe Publishing Ltd
18 Marcham Road
Abingdon
Oxon OX14 1AA
United Kingdom

www.radcliffepublishing.com

Electronic catalogue and worldwide online ordering facility.

British Library Cataloguing in Publication Data

A catalogue record for this book is available from the British Library.

ISBN-13: 978 184619 373 6

The paper used for the text pages of this book
is FSC certified. FSC (The Forest Stewardship
Council) is an international network to promote
responsible management of the world's forests.

FSC

Mixed Sources
Product group from well-managed
forests and other controlled sources

Cert no. SA-COC-001530
www.fsc.org
© 1996 Forest Stewardship Council

Typeset by Pindar New Zealand, Auckland, New Zealand
Printed and bound by Hobbs the Printers, Totton, Hants, UK

Contents

Foreword

Psychiatry as a discipline has a multi-faceted approach to diagnosis and management of mental health problems. Using biological, psychological and social models for understanding human distress, psychiatrists can put together treatment packages treating patients in a holistic manner. Medicine as a profession owes to its patients and to society at large the best and most suitable treatments. The core function of the profession is to heal and doctoring. Medicine and psychiatry, both based on science, require the art of caring, using the principles of art in learning and teaching. Psychiatry and its specialties can learn about mental illness and society's response to mental illness from textbooks, but equally importantly experience these emotions from cinema, fairy tales, poetry, literature, drama, paintings and other media. There have been studies looking at the creative nature associated with mental illness, but more significantly art itself holds a mirror up to society. Looking at the arts, the progress or lack thereof, can be seen and experienced. Arts form a core of the human 'being' and 'feeling' and the way art reflects society varies according to cultural differences and also in response to cultural differences in visual perception.

Using drama, poetry, music or therapies allows patients to express their feelings in a non-threatening and sensitive manner. Both educators and students need to be aware of the role the arts play in life and society. There is a danger that with increased technical advances, doctors may turn into technicians. One way of avoiding this is to instil in medical students and trainee doctors the notion that healing itself is an art. Sitting with a patient, making sense of their distress, being empathetic in understanding both the symptoms and the person and alleviating suffering needs a human touch. For that, doctors need the soul of an artist and must be aware of the value that arts have for society and the individual. This book brings together enthusiasts who have put together a much needed and welcome volume which hopefully will attract the wide readership it richly deserves.

Dinesh Bhugra
Professor of Mental Health & Cultural Diversity
Institute of Psychiatry, King's College London and
President, Royal College of Psychiatrists
June 2010

Foreword

Scholars in the humanities believe that all knowledge is connected and that these connections best help us understand what it means to be human. The arts in particular, by invoking all the senses, present vivid, unforgettable glimpses of reality. They allow us to stretch our worldview to transcend time, the body, culture and social status. Music, painting and literature portray themes all too familiar to the psychiatrist (loss, love, conflict, redemption) but seductively insist that we use both hemispheres of our brains, the emotional and the analytic, to interpret them. Reading a poem or following the lines of a drawing demands that we pay special attention, that we embrace an aesthetic, unpragmatic sense of the world. If we then discuss our reactions to a work with our colleagues or patients, we will be reminded and then humbled that words and colours mean very different things to different people. Ambiguity and the multiplicity of meaning are not only to be tolerated, but celebrated when we contemplate art. These are indeed valuable lessons to professionals in mental health whose job it is to co-construct meaningful, fully embodied narratives with their patients. Our work as psychiatrists has become increasingly biological. Diagnosis (even on five axes) can become an anti-narrative, one dimensional act. We may have improved the scientific credibility and reliability of our work, but at times, run the risk of losing its soul.

The authors of this wonderful handbook provide a convincing argument that the arts are good for what ails us. Just when we think we've heard (or seen) it all before, a scene in a film or play can surprise, even defamiliarise us from what we think we know so far. We may experience joy, outrage, catharsis, but we are changed. We are also reminded that the arts allow us (as busy, sometimes burdened clinicians) to climb back into the human race. We can be just as moved or surprised as 'non-healers', yet are in no way responsible for 'fixing' what we've just witnessed. Nonetheless, our moral imagination is engaged. We are reminded that nothing human should be foreign to us in the work we do. We have just entered a world which may provide a metaphor, image or point of entry down the line to help us recharge our own creative imperative or sense of vocation.

This comprehensive work reminds us that for real learning to happen both thought and emotion must be activated and subjective experience honoured alongside intellectual rigour. The authors know of what they speak. They have each used a preferred (dare I say beloved) artistic medium to deepen personal reflection and to enhance their own creativity as physicians, teachers and therapists. Their models are clear, their suggestions practical, but none of the approaches you'll find here are reductive or simplistic. I encourage the reader to savour each chapter and then to seek out the recommended texts, films and images to deepen the experience. Try some of the reflective exercises and teaching strategies. You will be sure to rediscover something you have always cherished about the art of healing.

Allan D Peterkin
Associate Professor of Psychiatry and Family Medicine
University of Toronto
Head, Program in Narrative and Healthcare Humanities
Mount Sinai Hospital
Founding editor
ARS MEDICA: A Journal of Medicine, The Arts and Humanities
www.ars-medica.ca
June 2010

About the editor

Victoria Tischler CPsychol, BSW, MSocSc, PhD, PGCHE

Victoria Tischler is a chartered psychologist. She has taught behavioural sciences to medical students and psychiatry trainees at the University of Nottingham since 2002. Her research interests concern creativity and mental illness and psychosocial issues related to the mental health of women, children and young people. She has developed a number of humanities courses for medical students. She coordinates visual arts exhibitions on mental health themes and regularly gives public talks on psychology related to art. She is on the editorial board for the *Journal of Applied Arts and Health*. She is patron of Open Art Surgery, a medical student arts society and a board member for City Arts, Nottingham.

Contributors

Allan Beveridge MPhil, FRCPsych

Dr Allan Beveridge is a Consultant Psychiatrist at the Queen Margaret Hospital in Dunfermline. He lectures at the Department of Psychiatry of Edinburgh University and also at Queen Margaret College on the history of psychiatry, and on art and mental illness. He is an assistant editor of the *British Journal of Psychiatry*, where he edits the 'Psychiatry in Pictures' series and is one of the book review editors. He is an assistant editor of *History of Psychiatry*, where he is also one of the book review editors. He has over 60 publications, including seven book chapters, on such subjects as the history of psychiatry, ethics and the relation of the arts to mental illness. He has written about Robert Burns, Robert Fergusson, James Boswell, Dostoyevsky, Kafka, Edvard Munch, Iain Crichton Smith and Charles Altamont Doyle. In 2006, he was awarded a Wellcome Trust Clinical Leave Research Grant to study the early writings and private papers of RD Laing, which are held at the Special Collections Department of Glasgow University. A monograph on this subject is in preparation and will be published by Oxford University Press.

Matthew Alexander PhD, MA

Matthew Alexander is Professor of Family Medicine at the University of North Carolina School of Medicine and Director of Behavioral Medicine for the Department of Family Medicine at the Carolinas Medical Center in Charlotte, North Carolina. He has a long interest in the medical humanities and is the lead author and editor of *Cinemeducation: a comprehensive guide to using film in medical education*. Dr Alexander's articles on cinemeducation have been published in such professional journals as the *International Review of Psychiatry, Family Medicine, Families, Systems and Health, Annals of Behavioral Medicine and Medical Education*. He is a distinguished public speaker who has spoken widely in Europe and the United States on such topics as the use of movie clips in graduate education, spirituality in medicine and an integrative approach to couple therapy. He has a busy private practice of clinical psychology as well as an active avocation as a singer-songwriter. Dr Alexander resides in Charlotte, North Carolina, with his wife, Elaine and their two children, Ethan and Natalie. More information about him can be found at www.alexandertherapy.com.

Thomas Schramme MA, PhD

Thomas Schramme is Professor of Philosophy at Hamburg University. Previously, he was a Senior Lecturer at the Department of Philosophy, History and Law, School of

Health Science, at Swansea University. His main research interests are in philosophy of medicine, ethics, and in political philosophy. He has published papers in *Bioethics*, *Theoretical Medicine and Bioethics*, *Journal of Medical Ethics*, and *Medicine, Health Care and Philosophy*, and co-edited (with J Thome) the volume *Philosophy and Psychiatry* (Berlin: de Gruyter 2004). He has also written a monograph, based on his PhD thesis, on the concept of mental illness, *Patienten und Personen* (Frankfurt: Fischer 2000).

Femi Oyebode MBBS, MD, PhD, FRCPsych

Femi Oyebode is Professor of Psychiatry and Consultant Psychiatrist, University of Birmingham and National Centre for Mental Health, Birmingham. Professor Oyebode has published widely on the relationship between literature and psychiatry. His research interests include descriptive psychopathology and delusional misidentification syndromes. He is also a poet and literary critic.

Arun Chopra MBBS, MMedSci, MRCPsych

Arun Chopra studied medicine at Aligarh University, India. He completed his postgraduate studies and training in psychiatry at Nottingham University and was awarded the College's Laughlin Prize at Membership Examinations in 2007. He has worked as an Officer of the House of Commons and with the Culture, Media and Sport Select Committee. He is working on his first book *Shrinking* (Radcliffe Publishing), a reflection on training in psychiatry.

Emily Ferrara MA

Emily Ferrara is an Assistant Professor of Family Medicine and Community Health at the University of Massachusetts Medical School, where she has taught creative writing, mindfulness meditation, and doctor-patient communication. She has published and presented nationally and internationally on the power of writing to foster personal and professional development, and on creative writing as a form of reflective practice. Ferrara is the author of the poetry collection, *The Alchemy of Grief*, selected to win the Bordighera Poetry Prize, and published in bilingual edition (English and Italian) in 2007. Her poetry engages subjects intrinsic to the human experience and the transcendent, including themes of love, loss, personal and professional identity, the illness experience, death and dying, and transformation. Her poems have received recognition from the Society of Teachers of Family Medicine, the Worcester County Poetry Association, and the Massachusetts Center for the Book.

David Hatem MD

David Hatem is an Associate Professor of Medicine at the University of Massachusetts Medical School. At the Medical School he is the director of the 'Patient, Physician and Society' course, a two-year course that teaches the principles and practices of medical interviewing, physical examination, clinical problem solving and medical ethics, and he has recently been named as co-director of Learning Communities at the Medical School, which will be launched in July 2010. He co-edits the 'Reflective practice' column in the journal, *Patient Education and Counseling*, a column that publishes narratives focused on the practice of medicine. He has co-directed a creative writing elective for second-year medical students for the last 12 years, and has taught and published on the role of reflection and professional development of medical students.

Mariangela Demenaga BSc (Hons), MA
Mariangela Demenaga has a degree in Psychology and Design Studies and trained as an art therapist at the University of Hertfordshire. Her clinical experience as an art therapist lies in working with adult users of mental health, learning disability and personality disorder services as acute admissions, in the community as well as in forensic medium and high-security settings. Mariangela has a special interest in art therapy work with people with schizophrenia and related disorders and is a visiting lecturer in professional training courses.

Daphne Jackson BA (Hons), PG Dip (Art Therapy)
Daphne Jackson trained at Sheffield University. She practiced as an art therapist in child and adolescent mental health services, and subsequently a special hospital (forensic) before taking up her current post as Principal Art Psychotherapist in a psychotherapy department. She has a particular interest in personality disorders and the use of art media to bring internal experience into the outside world.

Rob van Beek BA (Hons) Fine Art
Rob Van Beek is a visual artist based in Nottingham. He was an art student during the 1970s, a period of intense theoretical debate over the future of contemporary art, and took away a lifelong interest in the philosophy, psychology and politics of art. He has always seen the informal cultural networks of his city as his natural 'home' rather than any particular institution. However, he has worked as a tutor in adult education and as a visiting lecturer to many art colleges and universities. Over the years he has been a founder-member of many artist-led initiatives, including The Horse's Mouth artists' group, the Contemporary Aesthetics Network and the Nottingham Artists' Studios Open Festival. He is currently an active member of Making Waves, a mental health user group that provides training, evaluation and research. He is an executive member of Art in Mind, a project that fosters the arts in mental health in the Nottingham area. In 2000, he contributed words and images to Penny Arnold's film *Insight in Mind* and is currently involved in the production of a sequel about mental health recovery. Examples of Rob's artwork can be found by searching for his name in www.artreview.com.

Theo Stickley PhD, MA, DipCouns., DipN, PGCHE, RMN
Having originally trained as a mental health nurse and a counsellor, Dr Theo Stickley is an Associate Professor of Mental Health at the University of Nottingham and specialises in arts and health research. He is also an executive director for City Arts (Nottingham) Ltd and leads the innovative Art In Mind programme, promoting mental health through community arts. He recently led the development and delivery

of the Open to All training programme for museums and galleries for the National Social Inclusion Programme. This has now been completed and at its launch in 2008 the then Secretary of State for Health, Alan Johnson, gave his keynote speech on the arts and health. Theo has over 50 publications, a number of which are related to arts and health research.

Kate Duncan MA

Having originally worked as a ceramics and art teacher for nine years, Kate Duncan is Creative Programme Manager at City Arts (Nottingham) Ltd and specialises in community arts and social inclusion. Her interest in working with hard-to-reach groups has also led her to teach in several prisons in the West Midlands. City Arts continues to specialise in the delivery of arts and health programmes and the promotion of mental health, namely through their Arts on Prescription service. More recently, she has been exploring research models in partnership with the University of Nottingham that evaluate the impact of the arts upon well-being, with an aim to strengthen research and evaluation within the arts sector.

Neil Nixon BSc (Hons), MMedSci, MBBS, MRCPsych

Dr Neil Nixon graduated from University College London Medical School in 1996 and became a member of the Royal College of Psychiatrists in 2000. He worked as a lecturer in psychiatry at the University of Nottingham until 2005. Currently, he is a consultant in psychiatry with academic interests in neuroimaging, affective disorder and cultural/historical presentations of psychiatric disorder.

David Dodwell MSc, MD, MRCPsych

David Dodwell undertook his undergraduate training in Medicine and his postgraduate training in psychiatry in Manchester, gaining a MSc, MD, and Membership of the Royal College of Psychiatrists. He has worked in East Anglia since 1993, first based in Ipswich, then in Peterborough. He has specialised in working with people with severe, long-term psychosis since 1998 and is currently Consultant Psychiatrist for the Assertive Outreach Teams in Peterborough and Fenland. His main psychiatric interests are in communication and the relationship between staff and patients. He enjoys teaching and contributes to the Nottingham special study module 'The Arts in Psychiatry' for medical students and the regional MRCPsych teaching in Cambridge. David's father was an art historian and his mother a music teacher; he studied languages at school and developed lifelong interests in music, particularly blues, and poetry as a teenager; on and off he has played guitar and harmonica, and has written poetry, some of which has been published. He completed an Art A-level in 2007. He is now combining his interests in the arts and in psychiatry by studying for an MA in Medical Humanities.

CHAPTER 1

Why use the arts to teach mental health and psychiatry?

Victoria Tischler

INTRODUCTION

Something is lost, as medical students move through their training. I have worked in medical education for the past seven years and have had the privilege of sitting on interview panels to assess entrants to medical school. The process is highly competitive with approximately 800 students interviewed for a possible 260 places each year. All have exemplary academic records. Most have impressive work experience, for example working in healthcare in a developing country, volunteering in a local hospice or working as a care assistant in a nursing home. They also show evidence of a range of artistic, literary, musical and dramatic skills. I was recently presented with a children's book that a potential medical student had written and published. Overall, the students are bright, earnest, passionate and committed to a medical career. Many express an eloquent and clear understanding of empathy even though they are in their late teens. For those who are successful in gaining entry, the commitment and determination remain, yet I witness an erosion in the passion and enthusiasm that brought them to the study and practice of medicine, to the desire to care for and work with others. It may be described as a dulling that sets in almost imperceptibly. Is this a function of the way in which we train our students, the content and volume of the work that they have to digest, a coping mechanism, or something else?

The medical curriculum is densely packed, leaving precious little time for any other type of study or personal development. Students are expected to consume and assimilate huge amounts of information. They must demonstrate a range of clinical skills and they are required to adhere to strict guidelines on personal and professional behaviour. In my institution, apart from protected free time on one afternoon per week, their timetable is full, with students regularly spending 4–6 hours a day in the same lecture theatre.

In addition to my academic role, I am a senior tutor responsible for the pastoral care of students. Many students enthusiastically discuss interests and hobbies outside medicine when they start medical school. As they progress with their studies, I note that these activities are often reduced or stopped altogether, students citing that they have no time, for example to read or play a musical instrument. The initial enthusiasm that students bring to their medical studies also seems to dissipate as they move through their training, being replaced with a coolly dispassionate detachment. This is not to say that students don't care; on the contrary, I am impressed by the maturity, sensitivity and commitment that most demonstrate at a relatively young age.

In a holistic sense, something fades along the way. As educators, we don't nurture the student's whole being as they are trained. This observation could well be generalisable to the training of other health professionals and to higher education as a whole. The erosion in the autonomy of many health professionals, the well-publicised scandals in healthcare, the introduction of student fees and the economic recession, all play their part in creating the current business-like climate. The idea that higher education is a developmental phase in which to 'find yourself', to explore new ideas, to politicise oneself, to learn about a range of subjects, not just the one you are studying, is perhaps less relevant as students become 'customers' seeking the best possible degree for their investment.

As someone with a passion for the arts, I have always used film, poetry, drama, visual art and literature in my teaching. Student feedback indicates that such teaching is appreciated. Recent research that colleagues and I have undertaken suggests that the arts can bring humanity to medical practice, can help students develop professionally, and can assist in coping with stress.[1] One domain that the arts may particularly nurture is the development of empathic skills.[2] Empathy has been shown to be of considerable importance in medical practice, for example to aid effective communication. Paintings, novels, films and drama can absorb us and bring us to tears of joy or sorrow. Such media facilitate entry into the worlds of others, to experience it and imagine it. Students with limited life experience can utilise the arts to imagine life from another's perspective. They can do this by engaging with a piece of music about suicidal ideation, a poem from a spurned lover, a story about pathological jealousy, or an autobiographical account of bipolar disorder.

Art highlights, emphasises and explores core elements and human emotions. This provides a relatively safe way for students to engage with difficult and painful emotions that may arise in mental healthcare, for example working with those traumatised by childhood sexual abuse and those who enact their distress through self-harm, suicidal ideas or substance abuse. Literary works can also raise ethical and moral concerns which are commonly encountered in mental healthcare practice, for example detaining someone in hospital against their will. In addition, developing an appreciation for the arts provides a diversion from the demands of study and work and for some, a lifelong passion for creative expression in one or several forms.

This chapter focuses on the experience of establishing a humanities course: The Arts in Psychiatry. Prior to this course, the medical curriculum in my institution contained no formal humanities teaching. A previous module in general practice which had included material on literature had been discontinued.[3] I began by seeking out colleagues with similar interests. This was an interesting and affirming process as I found that others shared a similar vision and enthusiasm. I also made links with organisations such as the Association for Medical Humanities and the Madness and Literature Network. This networking and support in establishing humanities teaching has been invaluable. After some years and much persistence 'The Arts in Psychiatry' evolved and has been enthusiastically received by medical students and colleagues alike. The success of the course has led to the development of other humanities projects focusing on art and anatomy and drama and clinical communication, plus a range of associated activities described later in this chapter.

Although this text is primarily aimed at medical educators and their students, much of the material is suitable for students and practitioners of other disciplines; indeed there is much literature that supports the utility of humanities training in other professions, for example nursing and psychology.[4,5] Throughout the text the terms 'arts' and 'humanities' are used interchangeably and include visual arts, poetry, literature, music, film, creative writing and drama. This introductory chapter focuses particularly on evidence related to the study of mental health and its practice and includes a 'how to' guide for those contemplating establishing similar courses.

WHAT DO THE ARTS BRING TO MENTAL HEALTH PRACTICE?

The study and treatment of mental health is fraught with difficulty. It is a major healthcare issue with one in four people experiencing mental illness in their lifetime. Other estimates suggest that as many as half the (United States) population will experience mental disorder.[6] There are often no overt physical signs to examine as there are in other branches of medicine, and the concept of mental illness itself continues to be contested.[6] This has contributed to a move towards a biological understanding of mental ill health and a preponderance of research studies which utilise imaging techniques to demonstrate what is occurring in the brain. Yet, what does this tell us about the reality of living with depression, anxiety or schizophrenia? When a person is seen in the clinic, hospital or at home, a healthcare professional can observe an individual but is reliant on verbal reports or a narrative account to make sense of their experience of mental distress or illness. This emphasises the importance of perception, subjectivity and interpretation in mental healthcare.

The humanities integrate spiritual, physical, emotional and psychological elements, all of which must be considered in holistic, patient-centred healthcare practice.[7] The combination of arts with medicine evokes the German idea of *Wissenshchaft*, a science that includes both science and humanities[8] and is compatible with the recognition that psychiatry is both a science and an art.[7]

Art with its revelatory power has the ability to 'reach and express the depths of human experience' (p. 802), of critical importance in understanding mental health.[9] Humanities assist with the acquisition of a shared understanding by focusing on patient and doctor perspectives. This is essential for the accurate interpretation of a medical history, particularly in psychiatry where many symptoms are socially constructed.[8] Subjective experience is crucial in understanding mental disorders such as schizophrenia[10] and this is where the humanities can contribute in its many depictions of the human condition.[11] For example, from a psychoanalytical perspective, art can be used as a route into unconscious processes,[12] and by engaging with music, psychiatrists can move beyond observation and categorisation to understanding the inner world of patients.[13]

Humanities teaching emphasises reflection and active participation which may be viewed as an anecdote to the reductionist and technical learning which predominates in mental health education.[5] This is true of psychiatry where there has been a shift in focus from the mind to the brain[14] and where biological models for understanding mental pathologies currently dominate. At a macro level, involvement in the arts can facilitate community engagement and hence 'learning beyond the classroom'.[4] Such community involvement has many benefits including engendering a sense of belonging and cultivating 'cultural citizenship'.[15]

HOW DO YOU ESTABLISH AND RUN A MEDICAL HUMANITIES COURSE?

Finding collaborators

This was an organic process that involved discussions with a variety of colleagues in health and arts faculties within and outside my institution. I have been both reassured and delighted by the high level of interest and willingness to be involved in teaching. Anyone who has had to organise teaching schedules will recognise the difficulties in engaging busy colleagues to do additional teaching. In fact, positive feedback has been received from educators with some describing it as the most rewarding teaching that they have been involved with. Also key is gaining the approval and support of senior colleagues who control and manage funding. Endorsement of the course at a senior level also transmits the message that the humanities are valued as an integral part of professional health training.

Finding material

A book such as this would have been helpful in devising the curriculum when I established my first course. I am indebted to my colleagues Dr Arun Chopra and Dr Neil Nixon with whom I established 'The Arts in Psychiatry'. We spent many hours discussing the arts and debating possible course content. We found that each had interests in specific fields so we divided the search for materials accordingly. I led on visual arts, Neil on music and Arun on literature and creative writing. I also turned to colleagues running well-established medical humanities courses at other institutions. Here, I acknowledge in particular Dr Paul Lazarus at Leicester University, Professor Femi Oyebode at the University of Birmingham and Professor Jane McNaughton at Durham University. All were generous in sharing materials, teaching plans and most of all encouragement and support when obstacles came my way.

Recruiting students

Like anything new, the course (one of a large number of optional courses in the clinical years of study) required promotion. I designed and distributed posters and targeted the student body in advertising and raising awareness of the course. The relevance to clinical practice needed to be emphasised, otherwise some students may have felt it less worthwhile compared to the more 'clinical' options on offer. Take up was initially slow, however the course is now popular with students and word of mouth is an important mechanism for ongoing course promotion. Previous students have been involved in teaching on the course, which facilitates valuable teaching experience and also provides positive role models for current students.

Teaching format and style

Based on advice from colleagues who run well-established medical humanities courses, I adopted an 'arts-style' mode of teaching which offers small groups (6–14 students) high participation and a student-centred approach. Student-centred learning is acknowledged to have benefits such as increased motivation and knowledge retention.[16] Having experimented with various staffing models I have found that pairing a clinician with an arts scholar works well. This ensures that we offer specialist humanities subject knowledge with applied clinical relevance. This means that I have been able to persuade enthusiastic clinicians with interests in the humanities to teach on the course, reassured that an 'expert' is teaching alongside them. Both contributors develop session plans and students are sent materials and instructions in advance of teaching so that they are prepared and able to contribute in sessions. Sessions are usually two to three hours in duration so that there is ample time for viewing, listening, discussion, reflection and rest breaks. The timetable includes plenty of free time for students to read, listen to music, visit galleries, undertake research and to reflect on materials that they are working with. Some sessions, such as music and drama, involve two to three linked sessions. The aim is to provide an opportunity for students to immerse themselves in the arts for the relatively short 4½ weeks' duration of the course.

Facilitating engagement

Students are advised that participation is an integral part of the course and will be monitored. This is made clear in the pre-course information and in the introductory session where the educational rationale is explained and the ground rules for participation are outlined. This ensures confidentiality so that all feel able to contribute. Active participation is encouraged and modelled by educators who paint, play music and act alongside students. This is often a big culture change for medical students who may be new to engaging in this way and who can require encouragement and reassurance at the outset and through the course. Social events involving students and educators are scheduled and have included a cinema trip with the film (on a mental health theme) chosen by students and a group visit to an art gallery. Such events facilitate discussion and cooperation and foster a sense of trust and belonging amongst the group.

Assessment

Although the course is not summatively assessed, the students must complete it to a satisfactory standard denoted by either a pass, borderline or fail assessment. Students are asked to research arts materials related to mental health of their choice and to present it to the group at the end of the course (*see* Box 1.1). Presentations have included topics such as: depictions of obsessive compulsive disorder in the film *As Good As It Gets*, pain and the artwork of Frida Kahlo, an analysis of depressive illness in Sylvia Plath's *The Bell Jar* and suicidal impulses in the music of Trent Reznor (Nine Inch Nails) in his album *The Downward Spiral*. Students are encouraged to be creative in their approach to this and some have presented their own artwork and read poetry that they have written. Prizes of book vouchers are awarded for the best presentations.

BOX 1.1 The Arts in Psychiatry: assessment

Present and describe the resource and its creator. You should incorporate visual, audio or other materials as appropriate. You should refer to mental health symptomatology where appropriate.

Discuss how the resource has broadened your understanding of mental health and mental distress.

Discuss your personal reflections on resource chosen, e.g. how has the material affected you? How might it impact on your future medical practice?

Evaluation and sustainability

The importance of providing evidence of the value of this type of course is clear, especially in the current climate of evidence-based practice and efficiency drives. A research strategy should be built into any new course structure so that evidence is disseminated and available to support the educational outcomes and to persuade funders as to the potential effectiveness of this type of teaching. Preliminary research suggests that students are highly satisfied with the course, for example stating that it increased their confidence, addressed losses related to the all-consuming nature of medical studies, and helped them to cope with the stresses of a demanding vocational career choice.[1]

Associated activities

The course has led to considerable interest amongst colleagues locally, nationally and internationally. I have been invited onto two editorial boards, become the patron of a student art society, and have been asked to sit on the board of a community arts organisation. I was invited to be arts coordinator for the Institute of Mental Health and this has led to the development of numerous art exhibitions on mental health themes, for example, identity and visions. I have been invited to commission artworks for a variety of conferences. I have also been invited to talk about my research and teaching in a variety of academic and public settings. Students have gone on to be involved in teaching (as previously described), published reviews and poetry, acted as exhibition assistants, designed publicity materials and presented at conferences and seminars. Research projects, for example exploring creativity and mental health and the psychological impact of art exhibitions, have also followed.

THE CHAPTERS

This book is based upon the curriculum of 'The Arts in Psychiatry'. Each chapter outlines a topic, discusses its application to mental health and psychiatry and makes suggestions for planning and/or delivering teaching, giving a list of useful resources, if relevant.

In Chapter 2, Beveridge sets the stage by charting the historical development of conceptualisations of mental health and psychiatry through their depiction in the arts and literature, illustrated with examples from the visual arts such as 'The Asylum at Saint Remy' by Van Gogh and key texts such as Zola's *L'Assommoir*. Alexander gives a personal account of how he has integrated 'cinemeducation' into his working day in Chapter 3, using it in educating students and doctors, and in the therapy clinic. He discusses how film can be used therapeutically and educationally, for example to illuminate moral dilemmas and to stimulate discussion about sensitive topics. In Chapter 4, Schramme describes the work of the psychiatrist and art collector Hans Prinzhorn. He discusses the contribution that Prinzhorn made by identifying the characteristics of so-called 'schizophrenic art' and how art may help us understand others' minds. Suggestions are made about how students can engage with artworks created by patients and what this may teach them about the mental state of the artist.

Chapter 5 describes the role of poetry in explicating mental illness in its depiction of difficult human emotions. Oyebode argues that poetry is also a valuable medium through which mental health professionals can describe their own experiences. In Chapter 6, Chopra discusses the benefits of using literature in teaching psychiatry. He uses examples of texts such as Gogol's *The Diary of a Madman* and Kesey's *One Flew Over the Cuckoo's Nest*, used to stimulate discussion on topics like mania and electroconvulsive therapy (ECT). In Chapter 7, Ferrara and Hatem discuss creative writing courses and the contribution that they can make to the development of reflective practice in the health professions.

In Chapter 8, Demenaga and Jackson outline the history of art therapy and use case examples to illustrate how art can be used therapeutically to reveal mental states and to work through mental distress and traumatic events. Chapter 9 provides a personal account of mental health as van Beek describes his experience as an artist, service user and educationalist. He explores the aesthetic properties of mania and psychosis and invites evaluation of these experiences from arts and philosophical perspectives.

In Chapter 10, Stickley and Duncan discuss the political and historical context of community arts and the contributions that they can bring to mental health education, as well as to individual and social development. In Chapter 11, I discuss how drama can be used as a vehicle for improving clinical skills and provide examples of ways in which acting devices can be used with students to deepen their understanding of mental states. The final two chapters deal with music of different genres. Nixon discusses the utility of music appreciation in teaching psychiatry and uses examples from opera (Britten's *Peter Grimes*) and from the lived experience of Schumann. The final chapter by Dodwell is devoted to blues music, its history, context, subject matter and delivery. He discusses similarities between the blues and medical consultations.

CONCLUSION

When I started developing 'The Arts in Psychiatry' much research was required. There was no key text to recommend or to source material from. This provided the impetus to write this text and I hope it will inspire, guide and encourage others to develop similar teaching and associated courses. The text is not a definitive guide to medical humanities teaching and mental health but provides guidance based on the successful teaching model that I, and others, have developed. The course and its development have been time-consuming and challenging at times. This is far outweighed, however, by the pleasure I have experienced in discovering, and in some cases, re-engaging with many wonderful arts resources. It has been a personally enriching journey, as I have learnt alongside my students, deepening my own understanding of mental health. It is to my students that this book is dedicated.

ACKNOWLEDGEMENTS

Professor Nick Manning and Gerry Carton at the Institute of Mental Health, Dr Theo Stickley, Professor Paul Crawford and Dr John Whittle at the University of Nottingham, Kate Duncan at City Arts, Dr Jane Falk-Whynes at the Centre for Integrative Learning and my colleagues in the Division of Psychiatry, University of Nottingham.

SOME USEFUL RESOURCES

Association for Medical Humanities www.amh.ac.uk
Madness and Literature Network www.madnessandliterature.org
Literature, Arts and Medicine Database, New York University http://litmed.med.nyu.edu/
The Science Museum www.sciencemuseum.org.uk/
The Society for Literature, Science, and the Arts www.litsciarts.org/
The Freud Museum www.freud.org.uk/
The Wellcome Collection www.wellcomecollection.org/

REFERENCES

1 Tischler V, Chopra A, Nixon N, *et al.* Loss and tomorrow's doctors: student perceptions of the value of humanities teaching (under review).

2 Charon R. Narrative medicine: a model for empathy, reflection, profession, and trust. *Jama-J Am Med Assoc.* 2001; **286**(15): 1897–902.

3 Hampshire AJ, Avery AJ. What can students learn from studying medicine in literature? *Med Educ.* 2001; **35**(7): 687–90.

4 Thomas E, Mulvey A. Using the arts in teaching and learning: building student capacity for community-based work in health psychology. *J Health Psychol.* 2008; **13**(2): 239–50.

5 McKie A, Gass JP. Understanding mental health through reading selected literature sources: an evaluation. *Nurse Educ Today.* 2001; **21**(3): 201–8.

6 Pettus A. Psychiatry by prescription: do psychotropic drugs blur the boundaries between illness and health? *Harvard Magazine.* July–August 2006. Available at: http://harvard magazine.com/2006/07/psychiatry-by-prescripti.html (accessed 5 May 2010).

7 Bolwig TG. Psychiatry and the humanities. *Acta Psychiatr Scand.* 2006; **114**(6): 381–3.

8 Puustinen R, Leiman M, Viljanen AM. Medicine and the humanities: theoretical and methodological issues. *Med Humanit.* 2003; **29**(2): 77–80.

9 Biley FC, Galvin KT. Lifeworld, the arts and mental health nursing. *J Psychiatr Ment Health Nurs.* 2007; **14**(8): 800–7.

10 Chung MC, Fulford KWM (Bill), Graham G (editors). *Reconceiving Schizophrenia.* Oxford: Oxford University Press; 2007.

11 Kerr LK. Essay review: The humanities reforming psychiatry. *Theor Psycho.* 2009; **19**(3): 431–8.

12 Rosen I. Otto Dix: appearance and the unconscious. *Psychiatr Bull.* 1993 Dec 1; **17**(12): 727–32.

13 Durà-Vilà G, Bentley D. Opera and madness. Britten's *Peter Grimes*: a case study. *Med Humanit.* 2009; **35**(2): 106–9.

14 Rutherford BR, Hellerstein DJ. Divergent fates of the medical humanities in psychiatry and internal medicine: should psychiatry be rehumanized? *Acad Psychiatr.* 2008; **32**(3): 206–13.

15 Parr H. Mental health, the arts and belongings. *Trans Inst of Br Geogr.* 2006; **31**(2): 150–66.

16 Brandes D, Ginnis P. *A Guide to Student-Centred Learning.* Oxford: Basil Blackwell; 1986.

CHAPTER 2

A brief history of psychiatry through the arts

Allan Beveridge

INTRODUCTION

We can trace the evolution of ideas about madness through the arts, which have mirrored developments as well as shaped how insanity has been perceived and treated. In novels, plays, poems, biographies and paintings, we have countless representations of the mentally ill.[1] This chapter will provide a brief historical survey, using examples from the arts to illustrate key episodes and themes. Throughout history, explanations about the nature of madness have veered between the psychological and the physical, between the spiritual and the materialistic: that is, between seeing mental illness as a disorder of the psyche or soul, or seeing it as a disorder of the brain. Over the centuries, many have tried to reconcile this apparent conflict.

The mad have always been with us.[2] Our culture reflects this: In ancient Greece, Plato lauded divine madness, while Euripides warned that those whom the gods wished to destroy, they first made mad. In the Bible, Nebuchadnezzar is rendered insane by the Lord. In Shakespeare, we witness King Lear, blind and mad on the blasted heath; Ophelia, losing her reason and drowning herself; and Lady MacBeth obsessively trying to wash imaginary blood from her hands. In Cervantes' great novel, *Don Quixote*, we find the eponymous hero, driven mad by reading too many books on chivalry and tilting at windmills. In the Renaissance masterpiece, *In Praise of Folly*, Erasmus takes a witty and ironic look at the craziness of his fellow human beings. A century later in *The Anatomy of Melancholia*, the Oxford scholar, Robert Burton examined depressed spirits and how to counter them. In art, we have the paintings of *Melencolia* by Albrecht Durer, *The Ship of Fools* by Hieronymous Bosch and the nightmare vision of *The Temptation of Saint Anthony* by Matthias Grunewald.

THE EIGHTEENTH CENTURY AND THE BIRTH OF PSYCHIATRY

However, psychiatry as a medical discipline only emerged in the eighteenth century. It was a child of the European Enlightenment, whose leading philosophers challenged the notion that human beings should be guided by divine authority or deference to tradition. Instead, individuals would solve their problems by the application of reason. In like manner, the mysteries of madness would be unravelled by medical science. In the second half of the eighteenth century, the Edinburgh medical school became the dominant force in Europe.[3] It held that the nervous system was the prime operator of bodily function, a concept that overturned the teachings of the Dutch school, which held that the vascular system was pre-eminent.

The age of nerves and melancholy

The eighteenth century has been described as 'The Age of Nerves' because the incidence of nervous disease was perceived to be increasing alarmingly.[4] Many eighteenth-century luminaries, such as Samuel Johnson, James Boswell, Robert Burns, David Hume, Adam Smith and Tobias Smollett suffered from nerves. The most famous popular treatise on nerves during the period was *The English Malady* by the Scottish physician George Cheyne, who advised that it was only the well-to-do who suffered from lowness of spirits because their nerves were much more refined than the lower orders.[5] Another physician, William Stuckley, felt that melancholy especially afflicted artists, poets and philosophers.[6]

The eighteenth century has also been called 'The Age of Melancholy' because so many poets of the period, such as Blair, Cowper, Gray and Young, were preoccupied with the theme of melancholy.[7] A key novel of the era was Johann Goethe's *The Sorrows of Young Werther*, which recounted the sufferings and eventual suicide of a young man. In his autobiography, Goethe remembered the cult of melancholic self-absorption which characterised the period of the novel's publication. Speaking of the popularity of the work of the English poets of melancholy, Goethe writes:

> These earnest poems, which undermined human nature, were the favourites that we chose above all the others, one seeking the lighter elegiac lament, which accorded with his temper, another the burdensome, hopelessness of despair . . . everyone believed that he had the right to be as melancholy as the Prince of Denmark . . .[8]

In the *Lives of the English Poets*, Samuel Johnson catalogued the woes that befell the lot of the poet: Sir John Denham became temporarily insane; John Gay was often sunk low in spirits; Jonathan Swift went mad in his last years; and William Collins suffered from bouts of insanity. In addition, Milton was blind, Matthew Prior was deaf, the Earl of Rochester died prematurely from a life of dissipation, Richard Savage led an irregular life and expired in prison, while many others struggled with poverty and neglect.[9] Johnson's book was a favourite of Robert Burns, who declared: 'There is not among all the Martyrologies that ever were penned, so rueful a narrative as Johnson's *Lives of the Poets*.

Burns' letters convey his own struggles with despondency, for example:

> I am groaning under the miseries of a diseased nervous System; a System of all others the most essential to our happiness – or the most productive of our Misery. – For now near three weeks I have been so ill with a nervous head-ach, that I have been obliged to give up for a time my Excise-books, being scarce able to lift my head, much less to ride once a week over ten muir Parishes.[10]

Some took a sign of a superior sensibility for being prone to low spirits. This was a sentiment which James Boswell examined in his column, *The Hypochondriak*. Boswell began by examining this statement by Aristotle: 'Why is it that all men who have excelled in philosophy, in politicks, in poetry, or in the arts, have been subject to melancholy?' Boswell comments:

> Aristotle . . . appears to have admitted the opinion that melancholy is the concomitant of distinguished genius . . . *We Hypochondriaks* may be glad to accept of this compliment from so great a master of human nature, and to console ourselves in the hour of gloomy distress, by thinking that our suffering mark our superiority.[11]

In the essay, Boswell does go on to undermine the notion that melancholy was *always* accompanied by superiority but he appears to have a sneaking sympathy for the idea nevertheless. While Boswell might have been tempted to congratulate himself and his fellow sufferers on being a cut above the rest by virtue of their heightened sensibility, Samuel Johnson, who was also afflicted with depressed spirits, upbraided Boswell. Johnson did not feel that melancholy conferred superiority and advised his biographer: 'Read Cheyne's *English Malady* but do not let him teach you a foolish notion that melancholy is proof of acuteness'.[12] In Boswell's great biography of his friend, we read their many discussions about low spirits and how to counter them. Johnson favoured stoicism, whilst Boswell felt it was good to talk. In his novel, *The History of Rasselas, Prince of Abissinia*, Johnson's hero sets out on an adventure to attain happiness only to find that such a state is largely illusory.

Insanity and the beginnings of moral treatment

While suffering from 'nerves' may have enjoyed some social cachet, being insane certainly did not. The Scottish novelist and doctor, Tobias Smollett, caught this distinction in his novel, *Sir Launcelot Greaves*, when he described this exchange between patient and clinician:

> Doctor, (said our hero) if it is not an improper question to ask, I should be glad to know your opinion of my disorder – "O! sir, as to that – (replied the physician) your disorder is a – kind of a – sir, 'tis very common in this country – a sort of a – "do you think my distemper is madness doctor?" – "O Lord!

Sir, – not absolute madness – no – not madness – you have heard no doubt, of what is called a weakness of the nerves, sir . . ."[13]

The visual arts and the asylum

In the visual arts, William Hogarth depicted Bedlam in his series of etchings, entitled 'The Rake's Progress', which charted the downfall of Tom Rakewell whose dissolute life leads to his eventual incarceration in the London madhouse (*see* Plate 1).[14] There is the strong implication that madness is the result of moral weakness, although Hogarth was also pointing to the madness of society as a whole. In the nineteenth century, George Cruikshank was to pay homage to Hogarth's work by etching his own moral tale in which alcohol excess is shown to end in madness and suicide. The end of the eighteenth century saw the building of public asylums, although private madhouses and some institutions for the insane, such as London's Bethlem hospital and church-run asylums in Spain were in existence before this.

A powerful image of the new discipline of psychiatry was Robert-Fleury's painting of the great French alienist, Philippe Pinel, striking off the chains from a female inmate of the Salpetriere in Paris at the time of the French Revolution. Although it is unlikely this incident occurred quite as the painting portrayed it, Pinel did remove physical restraints from the insane and strove to bring more sensitivity to the doctor-patient encounter. In benign accounts of the history of psychiatry, his work is seen as ushering in a new era of humane treatment of the mentally ill. Rather than employing coercion, Pinel and like-minded clinicians would take a psychological approach that was christened 'moral treatment'. This would involve treating patients with respect, rewarding good behaviour and ensuring that they were provided with occupation and activities to retrain their disordered minds. Moral treatment was championed by the Tuke family at the York Retreat, which was to act as a model for other asylums throughout Europe.

Michel Foucault: madness and civilisation

This somewhat sunny view of the evolution of psychiatry was challenged by Michel Foucault in his 1961 book, *Madness and Civilisation*.[15] Foucault contended that the new discipline had actually introduced more sophisticated forms of control. Instead of chains, more subtle ways of restraining the mad were developed: patients were induced to construct their own 'chains', but these were mental in origin and served to constrict self-expression or any deviance from bourgeois ideas of decorum – they were, to quote the words of William Blake, 'mind-forg'd manacles'. By these means, Foucault argued, 'the voice of unreason' was silenced. Interestingly, he suggested that the voice of unreason could still be heard in those artists who had gone over the edge of sanity: Friederich Holderlin, Friederich Nietzsche, Gerard de Nerval, Vincent Van Gogh and Antonin Artaud.

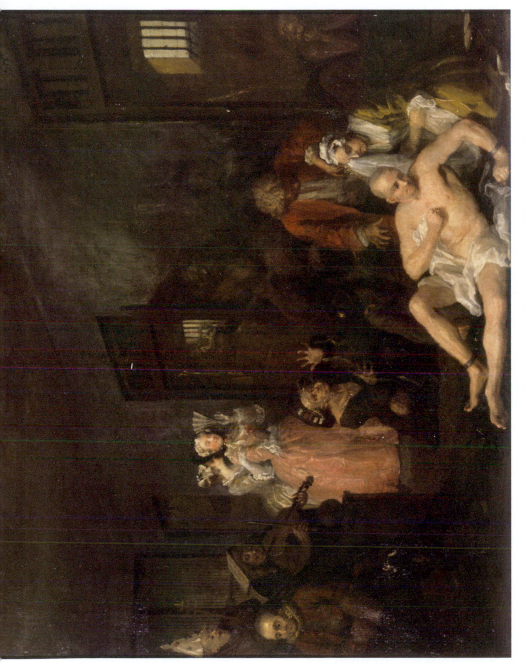

Plate 1: 'The Madhouse' from *The Rake's Progress* by William Hogarth. Reproduced by courtesy of the Trustees of Sir John Soane's Museum.

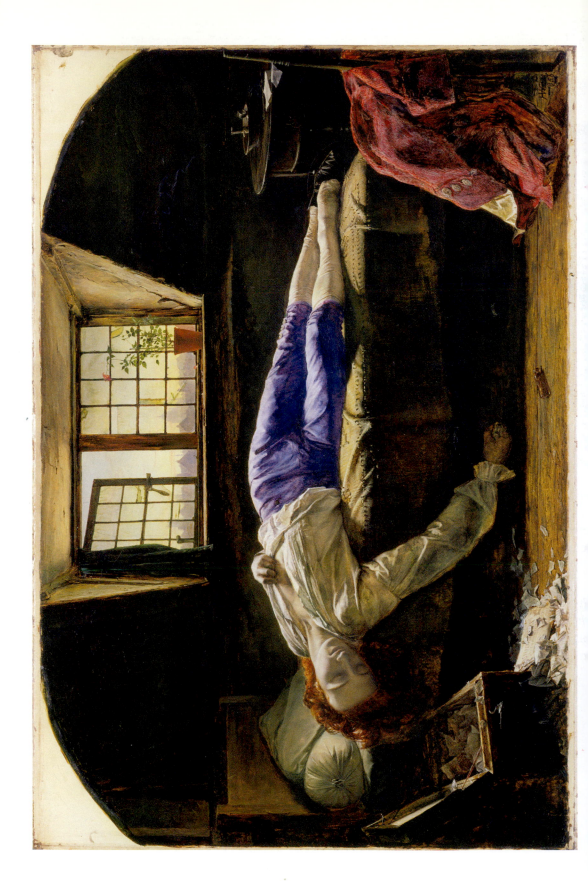

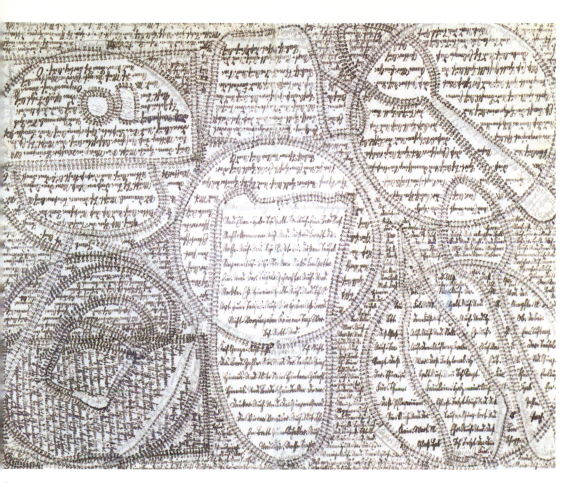

ove: *Plate 3*: Barbara Suckfüll. *Untitled*
ncil and pen on file paper).
produced with the kind permission of
nmlung Prinzhorn.

ht: *Plate 4*: August Klett. *Playful-decorative*
rk (water colour).
produced with the kind permission of
nmlung Prinzhorn.

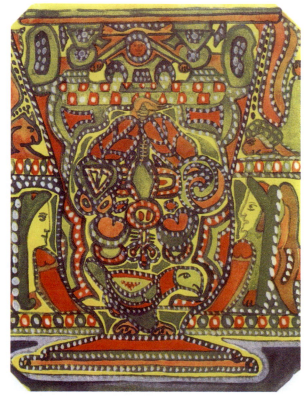

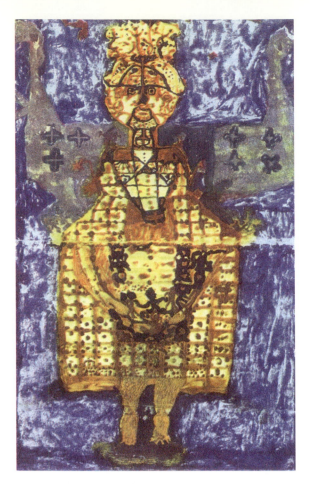

Plate 5: Hermann Beehle. *Sacramental (Idolatrous) Figure?* (water colour). Reproduced with the kind permission of Sammlung Prinzhorn.

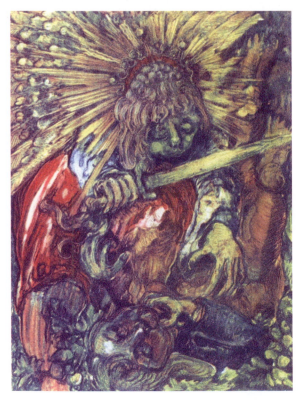

Plate 6: Franz Karl Bühler. *The Avenging Ang* (crayon).
Reproduced with the kind permission of Sammlung Prinzhorn.

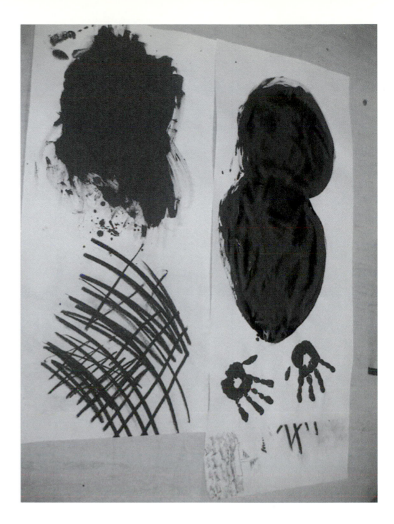

Right: Plate 7: Emotions find expression in fluid media.

Below: Plate 8: Jay with associated voices.

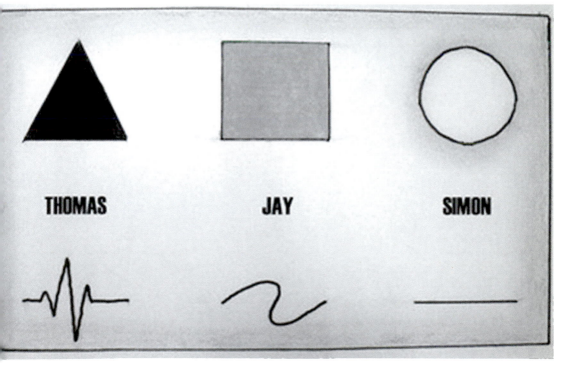

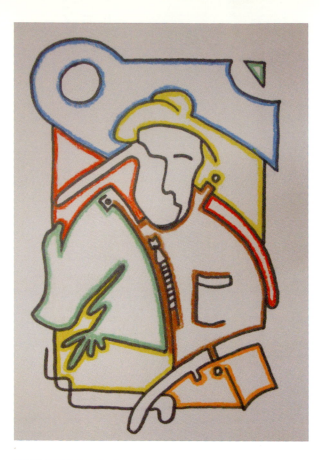

Plate 9: 'Thomas' in abstracted form.

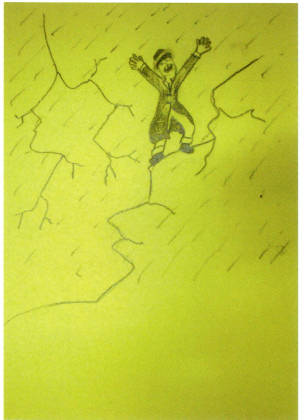

Plate 10: 'Thomas' enjoys the storm.

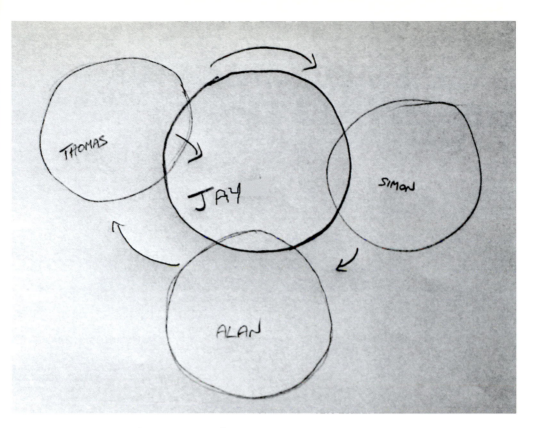

Plate 11: Jay with voices beginning to integrate.

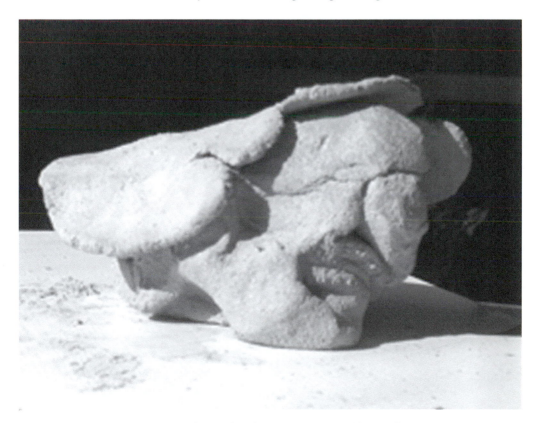

Plate 12: 'Grandma's pancake on Dad's head'.

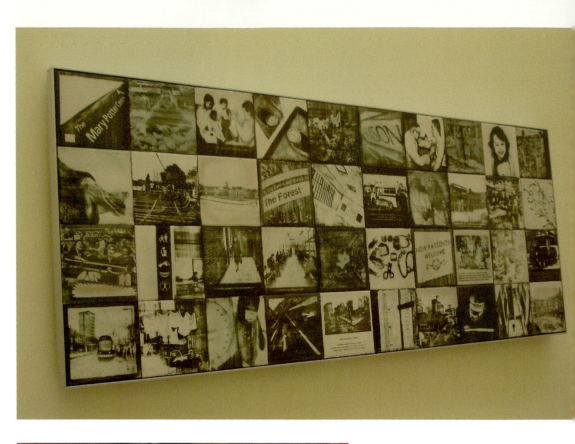

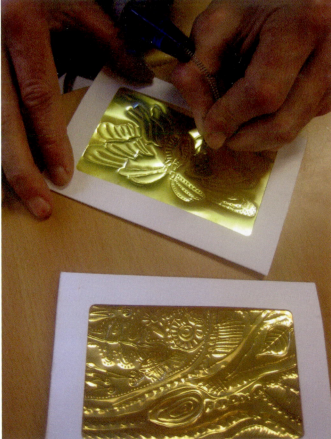

Above: Plate 13: Project delivered by City Arts at the Mary Potter Centre Nottingham involving centre staff, women's refugee and asylum seeker group and the local community.

Left: Plate 14: Participants taking part in the Arts on Prescription programme at City Arts, Nottingham

THE NINETEENTH CENTURY

The growth of the asylum

During the nineteenth century, asylums were erected throughout Europe. Novelists began to write about the newly built institutions, dubbed 'museums of madness' by the historian, Andrew Scull.[16] The asylums were often portrayed in novels as wicked places where perfectly sane people could be locked up by dubious doctors in exchange for large sums of money from relatives. Charles Reade's pot boiler, *Hard Cash*, was typical of this attitude, but more sophisticated writers such as Wilkie Collins also pictured the asylum as a nefarious abode, for example in his novel *The Woman in White*, which described the wrongful confinement of a young woman. Charles Dickens gave a more benign picture of institutionalisation in *Little Dorrit*, where Mr Dorrit only becomes mad *after* he has left the institution, in this case the Marshalsea debtors' prison. Dickens also offered an optimistic example of 'care in the community' in his novel, *David Copperfield*, in which mad Mr Dick is sympathetically supported at home by Aunt Betsy. This contrasts with Charlotte Brontë's depiction of domestic madness in *Jane Eyre*, where Mrs Rochester is described as a wild creature who needs to be shut away from polite society.

In Russia, the writer and doctor, Anton Chekhov depicted the asylum in his short story, 'Ward No. 6'. Here the asylum is a place of hopelessness where patients are neglected and the staff are corrupt. His predecessor, Fyodor Dostoyevsky, while rarely mentioning institutions for the insane, nevertheless produced work where a large proportion of the characters are mentally unstable, if not completely mad. This has led one critic to describe Dostoyevsky as 'the Shakespeare of the asylum'.[17] Russian writers have a tradition of being interested in the subject of mental disturbance. Gogol wrote *The Diary of a Madman*, in which the narrator thinks he is the King of Spain. Tolstoy's *Memoirs of a Lunatic* and *The Kreutzer Sonata* deal with insanity, while his *Anna Karenina* ends with the suicide of the heroine. In Goncharov's *Oblomov*, the hero is so afflicted with lethargy that he rarely leaves his bedroom.

The visual representation of madness

As well as writers, artists also explored mental disturbance. Francisco Goya produced two pictures of asylums: *Yard with Lunatics* and *The Madhouse*. Both depict the inmates naked and raving.[18] Swiss-born Henri Fuseli painted *Crazy Kate*, as well as works of imagination and horror, such as *The Nightmare*. William Blake, considered mad by many of his contemporaries, reproduced his visions in such works as *The Ghost of a Flea*. The French painter, Theodore Gericault, best known for his masterpiece, *The Raft of the Medusa*, painted portraits of the mentally ill and was guided by the theory of physiognomy, which held that the facial appearance reflected the underlying mental condition. Van Gogh spent time as a patient in mental hospitals, which he documented in *Men's Ward at Arles* and *The Asylum at Saint Remy*. He also portrayed his clinician, Dr Paul Gachet, who looked after him in his last months and was a patron of the arts. Charles Altamont Doyle, the father of Arthur Conan Doyle, sketched pictures relating to his stay in Montrose Asylum. The Pre-Raphaelite painter,

John Everett Millais portrayed the suicide of Ophelia, while his fellow Pre-Raphaelite, Henry Wallis depicted *The Death of Chatterton*, the eighteenth-century poet who poisoned himself (*see* Plate 2). Both pictures made an impact with the public and reflected the Romantic fascination with tragic youth. At the end of the nineteenth century the Norwegian artist, Edvard Munch produced pictures of anguish, such as *The Scream, Angst* and *Melancholy*. Munch had a psychotic breakdown, induced by his heavy alcohol intake, and received psychiatric help. Munch painted his psychiatrist, Dr Jacobsen and commented: 'I have put him in the flames of hell. He stands looking down as a pope upon his white-clad nurses, and us, the pale, sick ones'.[19] Unease about medical authority was expressed by Georg Buchner in his play, *Woyzeck*, in which a doctor experiments on a mental patient with no regard for the moral consequences and provokes his patient to commit murder. Disquiet about the abuse of medical science was also explored in Mary Shelley's *Frankenstein*, in which a doctor creates a homicidal being.

Darwin and degeneration theory

The latter half of the nineteenth century saw pessimism develop about the treatment of the insane. Asylums had been built in the belief that they would bring about recovery and amelioration of mental disturbance. However, as the century wore on, the number of admissions continued to increase, and the asylums silted up with patients with severe and incurable brain diseases, such as general paralysis of the insane. Faith in the principles of moral treatment, which in any case was difficult to implement in these 'gigantic' asylums, waned as Darwinian theory and notions of 'degeneration' began to have an impact. Such theories, as interpreted by nineteenth-century alienists like Henry Maudsley, seemed to suggest a grim prognosis of inevitable decline for asylum inmates.

Darwin's work had a profound effect on Victorian culture in general. Novelists, such as Thomas Hardy, George Eliot and Samuel Butler, responded to *The Origin of the Species* and its message that evolution proceeded impersonally and at random. As Gillian Beers has observed:

> One of the persistent impulses in interpreting evolutionary theory has been to domesticate it, to colonise it with human meaning, to bring man back to the centre of its intent. Novelists with their particular preoccupation with human behaviour in society, have recast Darwin's ideas in a variety of ways to make them seem to single out man.[20]

Darwin, himself, suffered from a range of obscure ailments, the precise nature of which has led to a welter of scholarly speculation. Darwin is often seen as a 'hypochondriac', using his symptoms as a way to avoid engaging with others or facing the uproar that his theories eventually provoked.[21]

Degeneration

The concept of degeneration developed as a consequence of evolutionary theory. The advocates of degeneration were primarily influenced by Darwin, but also by Jean-

Baptiste Lamarck, who maintained that acquired characteristics (whether positive or negative) could be passed on to succeeding generations. Degeneration theory was promulgated in France by J Moreau de Tours, Benedict Augustin Morel and Valentin Magnan; and in Britain by Henry Maudsley.[22] Although there were differences of emphasis, these clinicians broadly held that society was vulnerable to the physical and mental decline of its citizens. Part of the evidence of this decline was said to be found in the increasing numbers of insanity and cases of alcoholism, which were filling up the asylums. Degeneration theory held that mental disturbance became progressively more severe as it was passed down the generations. The French novelist Emile Zola was influenced by degeneration theory and, in *L'Assommoir* he depicted the decline of Gervaise, a working-class woman whose family sinks into poverty and squalor as a result of alcoholism.[23] Her husband is admitted to Saint Anne's asylum and a 'specialist' (whom Zola apparently modelled on Valentin Magnan) interrogates Gervaise about the family history of drinking.

> . . . he started to question her, rather roughly, like a policeman.
> "Did this man's father drink?"
> "Yes, Monsieur, a little, like everyone else . . . He was killed when he fell off a roof one day when he'd been having a few."
> "And did his mother drink?"
> "Lord, Monsieur, like everyone does you know, just a drop now and again . . . Oh, it's a very good family! There was a brother who died very young, from convulsions."
> The doctor stared at her with his piercing gaze. He continued in his rough voice:
> "And you, d'you drink too?"
> Gervaise stammered a denial, swearing it was the truth with her hand on her heart.
> "You do drink! Watch out, just look at where drink lands you . . . Sooner or later you'll die like this!"

Degeneration theory also affected how artists were perceived. As Porter has observed, Romantic artists, like Blake, Holderlin and Schumann had gloried in their transcendental visions or seen madness as the cost of creativity.[24] Degenerationist psychiatrists, such as Cesare Lombroso from Italy and Theo Hyslop from England, contended that the madness of artists was a sign of their flawed humanity and general inadequacy. In the 1890s, the Hungarian physician, Max Nordeau published *Degeneration*, in which he described modern artists, writers and musicians as 'degenerates', although George Bernard Shaw was to counter such theories in *The Sanity of Art*.

The fin de siècle: medicine and the arts

The *fin de siecle* was haunted by fears of degeneration but, as Mark Micale has shown, it also witnessed a great interplay between the arts and science.[25] A figure who typified this cross-cultural exchange was the French neurologist, Jean-Martin Charcot, who held court in the Salpetriere, where he demonstrated the signs and symptoms of hysteria to an audience that included the young Sigmund Freud. The theatrical nature of these demonstrations was caught in the famous painting by Andre Brouillet. During the evenings, Charcot, who was interested in art and photography, held *soirees* to which artists, writers and physicians flocked. Marcel Proust, the son of a doctor, was to later draw on Charcot's ideas about hysteria in his vast work, *In Search of Lost Time*, which also depicted depression, lethargy and nervous indisposition. Outside Paris, other figures combined a life of art and science. In Germany, Ernst Haeckel, the zoologist who championed Darwinian theory and is best known for putting forward the concept that 'ontogeny recapitulates phylogeny', was also a gifted artist. In Austria, the playwright and novelist, Arthur Schnitzler, had originally trained in medicine and specialised in psychiatry.

Nineteenth-century novelists took an interest in abnormal psychology. Robert Louis Stevenson's *The Strange Case of Dr Jekyll and Mr Hyde*, was only the best known of works that explored the phenomenon of split personality, a subject which clinicians such as Frederic Myers in England and Pierre Janet in France were exploring. Another Scottish writer, James Hogg had written about divided personalities some decades earlier. In his extraordinary novel, *The Private Memoirs and Confessions of a Justified Sinner*, the central character Robert Wringhim is plagued by his diabolical double and loses his mind. Hogg provides both a naturalistic and a supernaturalistic account of Wringhim's downfall and the reader has to decide whether he is mad or possessed by the devil.

THE TWENTIETH CENTURY AND BEYOND

The World Wars and the Holocaust

The twentieth century witnessed two World Wars and the Holocaust. The First World War gave rise to a new psychiatric disorder: 'shell shock'. Thousands of men had to be sent home from the front as a result of a disabling condition which rendered them unable to function. Historians have been divided as to whether this represented what would now be called post-traumatic stress disorder or whether it should be seen as a condition specific to the time and place from which it emerged.[26] Nevertheless, the episode proved to be significant in the evolution of ideas about treatment. Dr William Rivers, who worked at Craiglockhart military hospital in Edinburgh, where many shell-shock victims were sent, found that a kind of talking therapy based on letting the soldiers recount their experiences was more effective than physical methods. Craiglockhart received the war poets, Siegfried Sassoon and Wilfred Owen, an episode that was to be imaginatively recreated by Pat Barker in her novel, *Regeneration*. In France, the writer and doctor, Louis-Ferdinand Celine suffered a mental breakdown while serving as a soldier in the Great War and had to be admitted to a psychiatric hospital. He subsequently wrote about this in his classic novel, *Long Day's Journey into Night*, which described the futility of war and anticipated the central premise of Joseph Heller's *Catch 22*: that the authorities viewed a perfectly sane desire not to fight or be killed as evidence of madness.

The genocide which the Nazis unleashed during the Second World War had been rehearsed in the psychiatric hospitals of Germany some years before. Nazi eugenic thinking had decreed that there were 'lives unworthy of life', and as a result thousands of patients suffering from conditions, such as schizophrenia and learning disability were murdered in psychiatric hospitals. The lethal techniques which had been perfected to achieve the swift dispatch of the mentally ill were put to further use in the mass-extermination of Jews, Gypsies and homosexuals throughout Europe in the war years. The work of Franz Kafka, many of whose family perished in the death camps, is often taken as anticipating the Holocaust. Victor Frankl, a psychiatrist who survived the concentration camps, went on to write about his experiences in his book, *Man's Search for Meaning*. Frankl maintained that the fundamental concern of human beings was to find purpose to their lives. Albert Camus' novel *The Plague* was a response to the Nazi occupation of France and a meditation on human suffering. But, as George Steiner has asked, why was European culture, with all its glories of artistic and intellectual achievement, powerless to prevent the unimaginable horror of the Nazi genocide?[27]

Freud and psychoanalysis

By the middle of the twentieth century, the poet WH Auden was proclaiming of Sigmund Freud:

> to us he is no more a person
> now but a whole climate of opinion
> under whom we conduct our different lives.[28]

Even if one disagrees with his theories, it is true that Freudian ideas have permeated our culture. As Gillian Beers has observed:

> We now live in a post-Freudian age: it is impossible, in our culture, to live a life which is not charged with Freudian assumptions, patterns for apprehending experience, ways of perceiving relationships, even if we have not read a word of Freud . . .[29]

Freud has arguably had more influence on the arts than on psychiatry. Writers such as Virginia Wolff, DH Lawrence, James Joyce and Thomas Mann produced novels that have echoes of his ideas. In fact, Freud maintained that he had not discovered the unconscious – writers had done so before him. The Surrealists, such as Salvador Dali, Max Ernst and Paul Delvaux, were inspired by Freud and sought to explore the unconscious. They saw dreams, automatic writing and madness as a means of entering this dark and disturbing territory. They regarded madness as a state of absolute freedom – a state in which bourgeois law had no jurisdiction. In the first *Surrealist Manifesto*, the leading theorist of the movement, André Breton, who was also a doctor and had worked in psychiatry, wrote:

> The confidences of madmen: I would spend my life in provoking them. They
> are people of a scrupulous honesty, and whose innocence is equalled only by
> mine. Columbus had to sail with madmen to discover America.[30]

A few years later, Breton published an autobiographical novel, *Nadja*, in which he
described his real-life encounter with a young woman who was descending into psychosis. Here he did indeed provoke the confidences of the mad. The young woman,
the eponymous Nadja, formed a relationship with Breton during which she became
mentally more disturbed, ultimately being admitted to an asylum. In her last weeks
with Breton she completed a series of drawings, some of which were reproduced in
the novel.

The Surrealist view of insanity was essentially a Romantic one, in which madness
was seen as a process of liberation—a voyage of discovery to the unconscious. This
Romantic view was undermined by the fate of an artist connected with Surrealist
circles, Antonin Artaud, whose mental breakdown demonstrated that madness was
a terrifying and dislocating experience.[31] Artaud heard voices, developed delusions
about doubles and magical conspiracies, and had bouts of extreme withdrawal. He
spent several years in asylums, where he drew pictures and came to identify with
Vincent Van Gogh. Artaud contended that society was hostile to men of genius, lock-
ing them up in institutions or driving them to suicide. In his famous essay on Van
Gogh, he maintained that the Dutch artist had been 'suicided by society'.[32] Some
decades later, the radical Scottish psychiatrist, RD Laing was to claim inspiration
from Artaud's essay.

Therapy culture

In terms of psychiatry, Freud's work was never embraced wholeheartedly in Britain
and, although it enjoyed a long reign in America for much of the twentieth century,
it has been ousted by the rise of biological psychiatry, which is at present the dominant model in the English-speaking world. However, Freudian theory is the heir of
the multitude of talking therapies that we have today. The sociologist, Frank Furedi
has claimed that we live in what he calls a 'therapy culture'.[33] By this, he means that
ideals of stoicism have given way to the notion that we need to talk about each and
every problem we encounter, that we need therapy and counselling to help us meet
the demands of life. Will Fergusson has mocked this in his novel, *Happiness*™, which
takes an absurd look at our preoccupation with self-fulfilment.

Brain therapy

The twentieth century saw the search for physical treatments for mental illness and, in
the early decades, 'desperate remedies' were introduced.[34] These included lobotomy,
malarial therapy, insulin coma treatment and electro-convulsive therapy (ECT), of
which only the latter has survived to this day. Janet Frame, the New Zealand writer,
spent long periods in psychiatric hospitals and was given a diagnosis of schizophrenia. She received insulin coma therapy as well as ECT. She was also considered
for psychosurgery, but this idea was abandoned when she won a literary prize. The

American poet, Sylvia Path, who suffered from depression, underwent ECT and gave a fictional account of her experience in the novel, *The Bell Jar*. In Ken Kesey's novel, *One Flew over the Cuckoo's Nest*, the central character, McMurphy undergoes unmodified ECT and subsequently psychosurgery. Here psychiatric treatments are being portrayed as means of social control and punishment for behaviour deemed by the authorities as unacceptable.

In the 1950s, a second wave of enthusiasm for physical treatments led to the introduction of the antipsychotics, chlorpromazine and haloperidol, and the anti-depressants, amitriptyline and imipramine. The mood stabiliser, lithium carbonate, was rediscovered in 1949. This led one medical historian to brand the advances in physical treatments 'a smashing success'.[35] Biological explanations of human distress have permeated the public consciousness, and, for example, the American writer, Elizabeth Wurtzel titled her novel about her battles with depression, *Prozac Nation*. As Elliot Valenstein has noted in his book, *Blaming the Brain*, there is a trend to see individual misfortunes as secondary to brain dysfunction and thus in need of physical remedies such as medication.[36] The psychiatrist, David Healy, has described the psychopharmacolisation of everyday life and observes that increasing areas of human experience are being reclassified as pathological and therefore requiring tablets.[37] Aldous Huxley prophesied this development in his novel, *Brave New World*. In Huxley's dystopia, the population is administered regular doses of *soma* to keep them content, but the drawback is that people are deprived of their individuality and sense of responsibility.

Existential psychiatry

As well as psychodynamic and biological explanations of mental illness, the mid part of the twentieth century also witnessed existential approaches to the subject. In *The Divided Self*, the Glasgow psychiatrist, RD Laing argued that psychosis could be understood in terms of the individual's sense of ontological security in the world.[38] Laing was influenced by the work of the American literary critic, Lionel Trilling, who, in *The Opposing Self*, had argued that modern artists lacked the sense of being at home in the world, which their predecessors, such as Shakespeare had enjoyed.[39] Trilling took Kafka as representative of this tendency. Laing drew on this idea to describe the psychologically tenuous condition of individuals who suffered from schizophrenia. He combined continental philosophy with reference to such writers as Dostoyevsky, Beckett and Sartre. Laing was in fact steeped in European literature and his work was greatly enriched by his reference to novelists, poets and playwrights. In turn, Laing's work was to have an influence on writers such as Martin Esslin, Tom Leonard, Alasdair Gray and Doris Lessing.

Postpsychiatry

Cultural commentators maintain that we live in a postmodern world. The so-called 'grand narratives', such as Marxism, Freudianism and Christianity have lost their explanatory power. There is no longer one all-encompassing theory which fits all the facts. Instead, we have multiple perspectives on the world and no one perspective is privileged. In their book, *Postpsychiatry*, the psychiatrists, Pat Bracken and Phil Thomas, argue that mental illness is best approached from a postmodern viewpoint.[40] They contend that we need to be aware of the many different perspectives that bear on mental disturbance, especially that of the sufferer. In fact such notions predate postmodernism: imaginative literature contains many examples of texts that offer different accounts of the same topic. James Hogg's *Confessions of a Justified Sinner* has already been mentioned, but there is also Tobias Smollett's *The Adventures of Humphry Clinker*, Alasdair Gray's *Poor Things* and the novels of Dostoyevsky, described as 'polyphonic' by the critic, Mikhail Bakhtin, because they reveal a host of different voices, which overturn the conceit of an omniscient narrator.

CONCLUSION

This chapter has looked at the development of the history of psychiatry through the lens of the arts. By doing so, it has suggested that the cultural context has a major impact on how we perceive and think about madness. An acquaintance with art and literature can deepen our understanding of mental suffering.

REFERENCES

 1 Gilman SL. *Seeing the Insane*. New York: Brunner, Mazel; 1982.
 2 Porter R. *Madness: a brief history*. Oxford: Oxford University Press; 2002.
 3 Beveridge A. On the origins of psychiatry: the contribution of Edinburgh, 1730–1850. In: Freeman H, Berrios G (editors). *150 Years of British Psychiatry*. Volume II. London: Athlone; 1996. pp. 339–66.
 4 Porter R. *Mind-forged Manacles: a history of madness in England from the Restoration to the Regency*. London: Athlone Press; 1987.
 5 Cheyne G. *The English Malady: or a treatise of nervous diseases of all kinds as spleen, vapours, lowness of spirits, hypochondriacal, and hysterical distempers, etc.* London: Strahan; 1733.
 6 Stuckley W. *Of the Spleen: its description and history*. London, for the author; 1723.
 7 Moore CA. *Backgrounds of English Literature. 1700–1760*. Minneapolis: University of Minnesota Press; 1953.
 8 Goethe. *Autobiography*. Quoted in the introduction to *The Sorrows of Young Werther* by Johann Wolfgang Goethe (translated by William Rose). London: The Scholartis Press; 1929.
 9 Johnson S. *Lives of the English Poets*. London: Dent; 1968 (originally published, 1779–81).
10 Ross Roy G (editor). *The Letters of Robert Burns. Volume 1, 1780–1789*. Oxford: Clarendon Press; 1985.
11 Bailey M (editor). *Boswell's Column*. London: William Kimber; 1951.
12 Boswell J. *Life of Johnson*. Oxford: Oxford University Press; 1980.
13 Smollett T. *The Life and Adventures of Sir Launcelot Greaves*. London: Oxford University Press; 1973.
14 MacGregor J. *The Discovery of the Art of the Insane*. Princeton: Princeton University Press; 1989.

15 Foucault M. *Madness and Civilisation: a history of insanity in the age of reason* (translated by R. Howard). London: Tavistock; 1965 (originally published in French, 1961).

16 Scull A. *Museums of Madness: the social organisation of insanity in nineteenth-century England*. London: Allen Lane; 1979.

17 Appignanesi L. *Mad, Bad and Sad: a history of women and the mind doctors from 1800 to the present*. London: Virago; 2008.

18 Hughes R. *Goya*. London: Harvill Press; 2003.

19 Prideaux S. *Edvard Munch: behind the scream*. New Haven and London: Yale University Press; 2005.

20 Beers G. *Darwin's Plots: evolutionary narrative in Darwin, George Eliot and nineteenth-century fiction*. London: Routledge and Kegan Paul; 1983.

21 Dillon B. *Tormented Hope: nine hypochondriac lives*. Dublin: Penguin Ireland; 2009.

22 Pick D. *Faces of Degeneration: a European disorder, c.1848–c.1914*. Cambridge: Cambridge University Press; 1989..

23 Zola E. *L'Assommoir* (translated by Margaret Mauldon). Oxford: Oxford University Press; 1995. Originally published in 1877.

24 Porter R. *Madness: a brief history*. Oxford: Oxford University Press; 2002.

25 Micale M. Two cultures revisited: the case of the *fin de siecle*. In: Bivins R, Pickstone JV (editors). *Medicine, Madness and Social History: essays in honour of Roy Porter*. London: Palgrave; 2007. pp. 210–23.

26 Shephard B. *A War of Nerves: soldiers and psychiatrists, 1914–1994*. London: Jonathan Cape; 2000.

27 Steiner G. *In Bluebeard's Castle: some notes towards a re-definition of culture*. London: Faber & Faber; 1971.

28 Auden WH. *Collected Poems*. New York: Modern Library; 2007.

29 Beers G. *Darwin's Plots: evolutionary narrative in Darwin, George Eliot and nineteenth-century fiction*. London: Routledge and Kegan Paul; 1983.

30 Waldberg P. *Surrealism*. London: Thames & Hudson; 1965.

31 Barber S. *Antonin Artaud: bombs and blows*. London: Faber & Faber; 1993.

32 Hirschman J. *Antonin Artaud Anthology*. San Francisco: City Lights Books; 1965.

33 Furedi F. *Therapy Culture*. London: Routledge; 2004.

34 Valenstein E. *Great and Desperate Cures: the rise and decline of psychosurgery and other radical treatments for mental illness*. New York: Basic Books; 1986.

35 Shorter E. *A History of Psychiatry: from the era of the asylum to the age of Prozac*. New York: Wiley; 1997.

36 Valenstein E. *Blaming the Brain: the truth about drugs and mental health*. New York: Free Press; 1998.

37 Healy D. *The Creation of Psychopharmacology*. Cambridge, Massachusetts; 2002.

38 Laing RD. *The Divided Self*. London: Tavistock; 1960.

39 Trilling L. *The Opposing Self*. New York: Harcourt Brace Jovanovich; 1955.

40 Bracken P, Thomas P. *Postpsychiatry: mental health in a postmodern world*. Oxford: Oxford University Press; 2005.

CHAPTER 3

A day in the life of a cinemeducator

Matthew Alexander

INTRODUCTION

I have always loved movies. I grew up during the 1950s in New York City, a few blocks away from Loew's Theater, a huge movie palace with mezzanine, balcony *and* gilded box seats. This is where I saw such film classics as *Ben Hur*, *Lawrence of Arabia* and *The Ten Commandments*, as well as other, not-so classic, movies, such as *It's a Mad, Mad, Mad World* and *Three Coins in a Fountain*. I was lucky to live during a golden era of Hollywood when the 'moving' pictures and movie stars were, literally, larger than life. Currently, I feel quite fortunate to be able to incorporate this same awe and love of movies that I had as a child into my 'day job' teaching medical students and residents *and* my 'night job' as a psychotherapist.

Cinemeducation refers to the use of movies and/or movie clips to help educate undergraduate and graduate learners in psychosocial aspects of healthcare.[1,2,3] A cinemeducator is someone who uses film or film clips in this fashion. In the past 30 years, there has been an explosion of interest in this teaching modality. Fueled in part by the availability of movies on VCR, DVD and now the Internet, movies seemingly are everywhere and, very often, in the classroom. A recent edition of the *International Review of Psychiatry* showcased the international appeal of cinemeducation,[4] highlighting a broad array of topics teachable, in part, through popular cinema and including chapters on Bollywood and the Tamil cinema. This special edition contained articles on the use of movies to educate healthcare professionals about issues such as marriage,[5] intimate partner violence,[6] ECT,[7] addiction,[8] and psychopathology.[9] Other recent articles have shown how movies can help teach psychosis,[10] empathy,[11] core competencies in family medicine,[12] family systems concepts,[13] multicultural competence[14] and differential diagnosis in psychiatry.[15] Movie clips can be used effectively in lectures, small group discussions or role play.[16] Movies and movie clips have also been used by therapists with couples and with individuals, an approach called 'cinematherapy'.[17,18]

To be sure, there are limits to cinemeducation. The movies don't always get things right; for example, the depiction of schizophrenia in the film *A Beautiful Mind* erred by emphasising visual rather than auditory hallucinations which are more common in those with schizophrenia (the more recent movie *The Soloist* seemed to correct this mistake). Other times movies can evoke unintended emotional responses in learners (or clients) that need to be attended to.[19] And, of course, movies often paint with a broad brush and build on stereotypes. The skilled cinemeducator, however, is aware of these potential problems and can use them productively in the classroom by, for example, asking what the movie got right about a particular diagnosis and what it got wrong.

This chapter will highlight a day in *my* professional life, the life of a cinemeducator. All the applications of cinemeducation, which I discuss in this chapter, actually do occur in the course of any particular working week. I have, however, taken the liberty of collapsing them all into one day. Counter times and/or DVD chapters will be provided for all the clips used in Appendix 1.

MY DAY
8:00–9:30 a.m.

My day begins with a seminar to the Department of Oral Medicine, a graduate residency program in general dentistry, housed at Carolinas Medical Center in Charlotte, North Carolina where I am on faculty. I lead a monthly series of hour-and-a-half seminars in Behavioral Dentistry, which cover such topics as motivating patients, practicing self-care and dealing with difficult patients.[20] On this particular day, we will be talking about *hateful* patients. I base this talk on a seminal article by James Groves in which he describes the behavioral characteristics of four types of hateful patients.[21] The focus of the seminar is to use movie clips to help healthcare professionals *identify* Groves' subtypes early on in the treatment, *discuss* emotions such patients trigger in providers and *provide* tips for successful management.

My goal for this seminar is to focus on Grove's subtype of the 'dependent clinger', i.e. patients who are initially very submissive and endearing to their provider but gradually over time become more dependent, entitled and, sometimes, hostile. I use three clips from the popular film *What About Bob?* to lead the small group (which consists of eight or so residents, an oral medicine faculty member and myself) in discussion about this hateful patient subtype. In the first clip, Bob Wiley, a multi-phobic individual, has an initial interview with Dr Leo Marvin, a psychiatrist to whom he has been transferred (having driven his previous psychiatrist to quit the profession altogether). When the assessment part of the interview is finished, Dr Marvin makes a few recommendations to Bob. Bob's response is 'over-the-top'; he states that Dr Marvin, unlike other doctors, can really help him and that now he can 'be somebody'. Dr Marvin, who himself suffers from a moderate degree of narcissism, seems to bask in the praise. Groves refers to this part of the 'dance' between provider and dependent clinger as the 'honeymoon' phase. I refer to the interchange between Bob and Dr Marvin as the 'hook'.[22] The 'hook' consists of effusive and unrealistic praise and is a common way that dependent clingers manipulate their providers upon first meeting with them. *Knowledge of this dynamic can be an important clue to diagnosis.*

After showing the clip, I ask residents to share similar experiences with dependent clingers whom they may have treated in the past. Over the years, I have collected many written communications to oral and family medicine residents from such patients after their first meeting. In one, for example, the patient writes the following after her first appointment: 'truly angels were smiling on me the day I got to see you for a dental appointment'. In discussing these real life examples of 'hooks', residents are shown that this interpersonal dynamic is real and not just a Hollywood concoction. We then identify feelings of dread that accompany 'over-the-top' compliments from patients and discuss how subsequent visits with dependent clingers can often be characterised by emotions such as aversion, disappointment and, in some cases, hostility.

A second clip from *What About Bob?* is then shown in which Bob arrives unannounced at the town where Dr Marvin is vacationing with his family. In the scene, Bob first finds and then beseeches Dr Marvin with the following demand: 'I need, I need, I need, gimme, gimme, gimme'. This is the very best representation of neediness I have *ever* seen in the movies and illustrates powerfully the sheer depth of dependency common to *all* hateful patients. I then discuss with the group their emotional reaction to the scene and ways to effectively set boundaries with dependent clingers.

In a third scene, Dr Marvin attempts to *kill* Bob by tying him up, attaching dynamite to him and setting a timer to go off after he has walked away. This clip is shown to underscore the importance of setting boundaries early in the doctor-patient relationship so as to prevent just such a build up of intense negative feelings in the provider towards the dependent clinger.

10:00–12:00 p.m.

My day continues with a small group discussion with four third-year medical students who are doing a six-week rotation with the Department of Family Medicine at the Carolinas Medical Center. As part of this rotation, the students are expected to choose a chronic illness and conduct an in-depth home visit with a patient having this disease. The students are then expected later in the month to present the patient to the group along with information about the patient's family, relevant psychosocial aspects of his or her situation and current biomedical guidelines for effective treatment. I co-lead today's discussion with a physician faculty colleague.

To help model what we expect from the students, we use a case example of 'Gilbert', a young patient with chronic back pain.[23] We base the case on 21-year-old Gilbert, the lead character in the movie *What's Eating Gilbert Grape*. We initially give some general background on Gilbert, who works as a stocker in a grocery store, is the sole support for his family and presents chronic back pain symptoms to his doctor (an elaboration on the truth used by my co-facilitator and me to tie this character to a chronic illness). After this brief introduction, we ask the students to provide hypotheses for Gilbert's back pain. These are usually biomedical.

We then show the opening clip from the movie in which Gilbert, in a flat tone of voice, introduces us to his dysfunctional family. We ask the students to co-construct a genogram of the family. The genogram is a family assessment tool, which is required for the students to complete with their chronic illness patient.[24] As we construct the genogram, we discuss examples of family systems concepts such as over-functioning, differentiation and family life cycle which are demonstrated in the clip and which may be useful to the students as they prepare their own chronic illness project. We then ask the students to provide new hypotheses about Gilbert's back pain which now include psychological factors such as depression and psychosomatic factors related to his dysfunctional family situation. Finally, we co-construct a treatment plan for Gilbert that addresses his chronic pain from a bio-psycho-social-spiritual perspective.[25] Our goal is to provide a fun means of teaching family systems medicine to medical students and, in the process, model for them an exemplar chronic illness presentation.

12:30–1:30 p.m

I am now scheduled to give a large group lecture to about 30 family medicine residents and attending physicians on the topic of professional burnout. To facilitate this discussion, I first provide a handout with common symptoms of burnout. I then show a clip from the movie *The Hospital* in which George C Scott plays Dr Bock, a newly separated, chief surgeon at an inner-city hospital who rails against medicine and his unfulfilled dreams during an alcoholic rant.

After showing this powerful clip, I ask the residents to identify signs and symptoms of burnout which they recognise in Dr Bock. These include:
➤ excessive use of alcohol and prescription drugs
➤ lack of self-care
➤ disillusionment and cynicism
➤ fatigue and loss of physical function (i.e. impotence)
➤ inappropriate anger
➤ mismanagement of boundaries.

The lecture continues with participants sharing their own experiences of burnout during residency and co-constructing ways to effectively prevent professional burnout. This same talk would be equally applicable if it were given at any of the other eight residency programs at our teaching hospital.

1:45–3:30 p.m.

I now transition to the longitudinal second-year curriculum for family medicine residents which I also co-lead with a physician colleague in the Department of Family Medicine. This curriculum occurs every Tuesday afternoon and covers common topics germane to behavioural medicine (i.e. depression, anxiety, family issues and substance abuse). Today's seminar is on alcoholism. To help facilitate the discussion and set up a role play, we use several clips from the movie *When a Man Loves a Woman*.[26] The residents have been asked prior to this session to read several current articles on best practices in diagnosing and treating substance abuse in primary care.

We first ask why substance abuse is so often missed in medical practice; we inevitably discuss issues relevant to the physician (i.e. lack of education, fear of losing the patient, hopelessness about the diagnosis) as well as the patient (i.e. denial, fear of being told to give up one's substance of choice, fear of judgement, etc.).

We then show a clip from the movie in which Michael (as played by Andy Garcia) goes out of town and Alice (as played by Meg Ryan) comes back to her swanky Bay Area home early from a 'drinking' lunch. She staggers into her home, dismisses the babysitter, flies into a rage with her young daughter whom she hits and then falls through the glass shower door unconscious.

Immediately after showing the clip, we must first process the shock that viewers feel when they see the violence perpetrated on the daughter. We then use the clip to facilitate a discussion of common features of substance abuse such as:
➤ the prevalence of substance use disorders in women
➤ the co-occurrence of substance abuse and intimate partner violence
➤ the presence of shame and denial in substance abusers
➤ the ubiquity of substance abuse in all socio-economic strata
➤ the impact of substance abuse on the family.

Following this discussion, we show a second clip in which Michael is at the bedside when Alice awakens, post-fall, in her hospital bed. She is apologetic and he is *very* understanding, perhaps too much so. We use this scene to facilitate a discussion of codependency, covering the following topics:
➤ What is codependency?
➤ What are the 'appropriate' emotions one should have regarding a partner's inappropriate behavior while under the influence of substances?
➤ What is the prevalence of codependency in the helping professions?

After a short break, we then ask residents to role play an interview with Alice, with one resident playing the physician and one playing Alice. The resident playing the physician is given some background medical information about Alice and the resident playing Alice is given a general script, true to her character, from which to act. The resident playing the physician is then asked to screen Alice for possible substance use disorders and eventually confront her about suspected substance abuse.

Following the role play, we debrief by asking participants and observers to share feelings and observations about the role play including perspectives on how well or poorly it went. We finish with a general discussion of the rewards and challenges of working with patients having substance use disorders as well as tips for management.

5:00–6:00 p.m.

Now that my teaching day is done, I transition into my private practice of clinical psychology. Clients often mention movies in passing during their sessions which provides an opportunity to find out more about their preferences in cinema as well as emotions and meanings triggered by their movie-going experience. I will, however, sometimes push the proverbial envelope a step further and suggest that a client or couple view a specific movie at home to highlight certain therapeutic issues and facilitate discussion.[26] It is important, however, that I be respectful and knowledge-able about my clients' tastes in movies and I rarely recommend a movie that I have not seen myself.

I begin my evening clinic with a 17-year-old client, Melissa, who is seeing me for depression. A key factor in her mood disorder is her relationship, or lack thereof, with her dysfunctional father, an alcoholic, who lives far away with his own parents and who has, for all intents and purposes, abandoned her. At the end of our third session, I ask Melissa to rent the movie *The Wrestler* and focus her attention on the failed relationship between the father and his adult daughter. In the following ses-sion, she stoically describes her reactions to the movie and fights back tears. While her situation is not identical to that of the character in the film, she can identify with the extreme disappointment and anger that the character feels towards her father. She is planning to cut off contact with her father, like the character does in the film. We are, however, able to have a discussion of the pros and cons of 'cut-offs' with important family figures, and while she ultimately decides to cease contact with her father while she focuses on other concurrent issues in her life, she remains open to possible future reconciliation. The movie served as a vehicle to help normalise her own feelings and facilitate a discussion of possible choices she has in her ongoing relationship with her father.

6:00–7:00 p.m.

My final work hour is spent with a couple who are at a crossroads in their marriage; the husband, Bill, has just had an affair (now ended) and wonders if he ever even loved his wife. The wife, Joan, is devoted but confused. One of the dysfunctional patterns in their relationship (there are many) is that Joan is a 'glass half full' per-son and Bill is a 'glass half empty' person. In session, they play out these roles . . . she giggles and he looks glum. I wonder aloud if these personality differences have become exaggerated over the years, polarising them into exaggerated versions of their original selves. This is a similar dynamic as is portrayed in the movie, *The Story of Us*, which I ask them to watch before our next session.

On their return visit, I find, not surprisingly, that the wife identified with Ben, the happy-go-lucky Bruce Willis character, and the husband with Katie, the more respon-sible Michelle Pfeiffer character. The couple observed that the movie showed how, over time, Ben and Katie insidiously lock each other into roles that do not feel good but instead fuel and deepen the disagreements between them. They could identify with that process and wondered how they could, themselves, become less polarised. I suggested for the next week that Bill get more in touch with, and express, his 'fun side' and Joan get in touch with and express her 'serious side', a role reversal which they found challenging at first but ultimately helpful to them. While the movie didn't solve their problem for them, it allowed them to see their own pattern in another couple, thereby making it less threatening to identify and modify the pattern in their own marriage.

SUMMARY

Cinemeducation is a fun and effective way to teach students and residents about the psychosocial aspects of their work. Cinematherapy is an innovative way of working with couples and clients. As cited in this chapter, there are numerous resources available for educators and therapists to immediately implement cinemeducation and cinematherapy in their teaching settings and clinical practices. I hope that this chapter serves to inspire and energise a whole new generation of cinemeducators. However, while anecdotal evidence supports the value of these approaches, there is a need for more research in this area to demonstrate their value to students, patients and clients.

APPENDIX

Note: Times may vary slightly on various VC players.

What About Bob? (Bill Murray, Richard Dreyfus) – The 'hook' (VHS counter time: 0:07:11–0:11:40).

What About Bob? – The unannounced arrival (VHS counter time: 0:23:50–0:26:20).

What About Bob? – Death therapy (VHS counter time: 1:26:37–1:33:22).

What's Eating Gilbert Grape? (Johnny Depp, Leonardo DiCaprio) – Introduction to the Grape family (VHS counter time: 0:00:00–0:06:13).

The Hospital (George C Scott) – Drunken tirade (VHS counter time: 0:49:50–0:57:20).

When A Man Loves A Woman (Meg Ryan, Andy Garcia) – Alice comes home intoxicated (VHS counter time: 0:30:40 – 0:36:27).

When A Man Loves A Woman – At the bedside (VHS counter time: 0:36:27–0:39:44).

REFERENCES

1 Alexander M. A review of the literature. In: Alexander M, Lenahan P, Pavlov A (editors). *Cinemeducation: a comprehensive guide to the use of film in medical education*. Oxford: Radcliffe Publishing; 2005, pp. 3–5.

2 Alexander M. *The Doctor*: a seminal video for cinemeducation. *Fam Med.* 2002; **34**(2): 92–4.

3 Alexander M, Hall M, Pettice Y. Cinemeducation: an innovative approach to teaching psychosocial medical care. *Fam Med.* 1994; **26**: 430–3.

4 Bhugra D, Gupta S, Lyketsos C (editors). Special issue on cinema. *Int Rev Psychiatr.* June 2009; **21**(3); 181–2.

5 Alexander M. The couple's odyssey: Hollywood's take on love relationships. *Int Rev Psychiatr.* June 2009; **21**(3): 183–8.

6 Lenahan P. Intimate partner violence: what do movies have to teach us? *Int Rev Psychiatr.* June 2009; **21**(3): 189–99.

7 McDonald A, Walter G. Hollywood and ECT. *Int Rev of Psychiatr.* June 2009; **21**(3): 200–6.

8 Cape G. Movies as a vehicle to teach addiction medicine. *Int Rev of Psychiatr.* June 2009; **21**(3): 213–17.

9 Datta V. Madness and the movies: an undergraduate module for medical students, *Int Rev of Psychiatr.* June 2009; **21**(3): 261–6.

10 Bell V, Laroi F, Raballo A. Humanizing the clinical gaze: movies and the empathic understanding of psychosis. *Fam Med.* 2009; **41**(6): 387–8.

11 Blasco P, Janaudis M, Levites M, *et al.* Using movie clips to foster learners' reflection: improving education in the affective domain. *Fam Med.* 2006; **38**(2): 94–6.

12 Alexander M, Pavlov A, Lenahan P. Lights, camera, action: using film to teach the ACGME competencies. *Fam Med.* 2007; **39**(1): 20–3.

13 Alexander M, Waxman D. Cinemeducation: using movies to teach family systems. *Fam Systems Health.* 2001; **18**(4): 455–62.

14 Alexander M. Cinemeducation: an innovative approach to teaching multi-cultural diversity in medicine. *Ann Behav Sci and Med Educ.* 1995; **2**(1): 23–8.

15 Robinson D. Reel psychiatry. *Int Rev Psychiatr.* 2009; **21**(3): 245–60.

16 Zagvazdin Y. Movies and emotional engagement: laughing matters in lecturing. *Fam Med.* 2007; **39**(4): 245–47.

17 Hesley J, Hesley J. *Rent Two Films and Let's Talk in the Morning: using popular movies in psychotherapy.* New York: John Wiley & Sons; 1998.

18 Sineta M. *Reel Power: spiritual growth through film.* Chicago: Triumph Books; 1993.

19 Campbell T. Foreword. In: Alexander M, Lenahan P, Pavlov A. *Cinemeducation: a comprehensive guide to the use of film in medical education.* Oxford: Radcliffe Publishing; 2005, p. xii.

20 Lockhart P, Alexander M, Pettice Y, Olson R. Behavioral medicine training in postdoctoral dental education. *J Dent Educ.* 1992; **56**(3): 190–4.

21 Groves JE. Taking care of the hateful patient. *New Engl J Med.* April 1978; **298**(16): 883–7.

22 The 'hook' is a term developed by Mary Hall, MD.

23 Alexander M, Waxman D, White P. *What's Eating Gilbert Grape:* a case study of illness. *Journal for Learning Through the Arts.* 2007; **2**(1): Article 13.

24 McGoldrick M, Gerson R. *Genograms in Family Assessment.* New York: Norton; 1985.

25 Hiatt JF. Spirituality, medicine and healing. *South Med J.* 1986; **79**: 736–43.

26 Alexander M, Pavlov A, Lenahan P. Lights, camera, action: using film to teach the ACGME competencies. *Fam Med.* 2007; **39**(1): 20–3.

CHAPTER 4

The quest to understand the afflicted mind: Hans Prinzhorn and the artistry of the mentally ill

Thomas Schramme

INTRODUCTION: UNDERSTANDING OTHER MINDS

Psychiatry differs from other branches of medicine insofar as it is concerned with patients whose affliction cannot be reduced to pathologies of parts of an organism. The psychiatric patient always has to be regarded as a whole person. The mind and its disorders are special in that they affect the very characteristics that make us persons, in contrast to mere biological organisms: we think, we feel, we value, we want, we intend, we imagine, and so on. Another important aspect of these mental activities is that they are invisible to other people. This is a problem, of course, that has riddled psychiatry for a long time and that has deemed it unscientific in the eyes of some critics. We cannot 'see' a mental disorder in the same way that we can see or prove the existence of a somatic disease. Psychiatry has often strived to follow the precursor of somatic medicine in trying to identify bodily afflictions that accompany mental disorder. But there are unsolvable problems for this approach, which have to do with the features of mental activities just mentioned. We simply cannot identify, say, the way a person feels by looking at the body, or the brain, for that matter. Although we know that the mind is somehow reliant on and related to the body, specifically brain processes, we cannot explain or understand complex mental activities by studying the functions of the nervous system. But to understand the human mind and its disorders is the very task of psychiatry. Hence, if somatisation of mental disorder does not work, there is a need to find other ways to understand the minds of psychiatric patients.

The problem of 'other minds', as it is called in philosophy, has a long tradition. We don't have direct access to other persons' minds; so how can we ever know what is going on 'in their heads'. In fact, how can we even be sure that they have a mind? Might they not be very complicated robots or, still more extreme, might they not exist at all and only be imagined in our own minds? After all, it seems that a person has direct access only to their own mind. So, the problem of other minds can lead to the radical idea of solipsism, the philosophical notion that only I exist. However, the problem of other minds is a very real and common one. It poses a severe methodological challenge for psychiatry. Historically, it has been tackled by behaviourism, and more recently by biological psychiatry. But these reductive approaches are doomed to fail, as stated earlier, because they don't provide the kind of knowledge needed when dealing with patients. Psychiatrists must aim to understand what it means for a patient to be afflicted by a particular disorder, on pain of lacking a therapeutic purpose. We will see in this chapter how an unlikely bedfellow of psychiatry, the arts, might open up new avenues to understand the afflicted mind. I will pursue this suggestion by introducing the exemplary work of Hans Prinzhorn.

But first, a word of caution might be in order. The topic of this chapter is art in relation to mental illness. There are a lot of (often wrong) assumptions concerning the relationship between creativity and mental disorder. Supposedly, people who are considered 'mad' are more creative than 'normal' people, and there are allegedly a larger proportion of mentally ill artists than afflicted non-artists. Some people therefore assume that mental illness can actually cause people to become creative, maybe even a genius. However, we know that people with mental illness do not produce more works of art than other people. On the contrary, the so-called negative symptoms of schizophrenia actually inhibit creativity. In addition, genius is usually not due to sudden outbursts of creativity but to long-term self-discipline. Mental illness is therefore a hindrance to the development of genius. Finally, mental illness is clearly not the cause of creativity, although it might boost achievement in patients who are already prone to creative work. For example, hypomania can produce long-term 'highs' and perseverance in people. The only connection between creativity and mental illness seems to be that divergent thinking, including uncommon perspectives on the world, is a common symptom of mental disorder. Mentally ill people often have a 'strong imagination'.[1]

HANS PRINZHORN, THE COLLECTION OF PSYCHIATRIC ART AND ITS DENUNCIATION AS 'DEGENERATED'

Hans Prinzhorn was born in 1886 in Westphalia, Germany. He studied a variety of subjects and changed universities several times. He first enrolled for art history and philosophy and received a doctorate with a thesis on Gottfried Semper's aesthetic principles at Munich University. In Munich, he then sought to make friends with artists, being a keen singer himself. His plans, however, to graduate in singing as well and to become a professional, failed mostly for reasons of ill health and also personal reasons – his then wife had become mentally ill. Prinzhorn embarked on a new career and read medicine at the University of Freiburg and Strasbourg University, where he graduated in 1917. This double qualification in the arts and medicine qualified him for his later work and scholarly research. More by chance than intention – on invitation of the newly appointed director of Heidelberg University's psychiatric hospital, Kurt Wilmanns, whom he had met whilst working in a hospital camp at the Western front – Prinzhorn became responsible for an already existing collection of paintings made by patients. In his short reign, between 1919 and 1921, he expanded it to include about 5000 samples of paintings, drawings, notes, letters and crafts made by some 450 psychiatric patients, mostly from Germany and Switzerland, the majority of whom were labelled schizophrenic. This assembly of items is known today as the 'Prinzhorn collection'. It is still based in Heidelberg and is now housed in a public museum.

In 1922, Prinzhorn published his study *Artistry of the Mentally Ill* (*Bildnerei der Geisteskranken*). In this book, he developed a theory of expression: a specific explanation of the sources and the formation of human creativity, and applied it to examples drawn from the collection. It is probably fair to say that his main interest was in aesthetic theory, in contrast to therapeutic practice, although an important purpose of his approach was to determine a better understanding of what it means to be mentally ill. Also, Prinzhorn did later work as a psychotherapist. The book was well received and quickly gained influence in the arts scene, especially with avant-garde artists like Ernst Klee, Max Ernst and Hugo Ball; Alfred Kubin even visited the collection as early as 1921. Later it became a kind of template for so-called 'Art Brut', initiated by Jean Dubuffet. However, the impact on artists was due less to Prinzhorn's theoretical considerations; admirers were fascinated by the paintings reproduced in the book, most of all by the works of the 'masters', as Prinzhorn dubbed them.

The Nazis, however, were less impressed. They exploited some of the items from the Prinzhorn collection for their infamous travelling exhibition 'Degenerate Art' (*Entartete Kunst*), which opened in 1938. Prinzhorn himself was deceased by then, although it should not be concealed that he had an ambivalent stance on the National Socialist movement and actually partially endorsed it in a series of articles in the early 1930s. Yet Prinzhorn died in June 1933 of pulmonary embolism related to typhus, so experienced the party in power for only a few weeks.

The notion of 'Degenerate Art' worked in two ways. It denunciated the artists of the then avant-garde as mentally disturbed by pointing out similarities between their work and items from the Heidelberg collection; and it established the 'worthlessness' of the artistry of the mentally ill – which eventually culminated in the claim of the unworthiness of the mentally ill themselves. Many of the patient-artists, for instance Franz Karl Bühler and Paul Goesch, were killed as part of the Nazi 'euthanasia' programme. The notorious psychiatrist Carl Schneider, successor of Wilmanns in Heidelberg, proved to be of vital importance for this programme. He was keen to supply the curators of the Degenerate Art exhibition with displays of sculptures and drawings from the collection, and published the article 'Degenerate art and insane art' (*Irrenkunst*) in 1940.

As far as the first purpose, the defamation of the avant-garde, was concerned, Prinzhorn proved to be far-sighted. In his book, in which he drew attention to similarities between expressionist painters and works of the patients, he stated:

The conclusion that a painter is mentally ill because he paints like a given mental patient is no more intelligent or convincing than another; viz., that Pechstein and Heckel are Africans from the Camerouns because they produce wooden figurines like those by the Africans from the Camerouns. (p. 271).[2]

THE 'MATERIALISATION OF THE SOUL' IN IMAGES

Prinzhorn's *Artistry of the Mentally Ill,* which he wrote in a very short period of time, was a major achievement and is still, to date, a valuable read. It combines in-depth studies of 10 patient 'masters', some of who were actually professional artists, with a theoretical analysis of the process of creation and expression. It gives evidence of a time when philosophical and psychological findings were still considered in conjunction. Prinzhorn calls his study a 'contribution to a future psychology of configuration' (p. 4),[2] but one might also say that it is a work of philosophical anthropology, focused on a particular aspect of being a human person, namely the aspect of expressing oneself in images.

The English title of the book is possibly misleading, as Prinzhorn was not concerned with the question of whether the collected paintings were really pieces of art, although he certainly considered many of them to be masterpieces. Rather, he referred to them neutrally as 'images', and the German title actually refers to *Bildnerei,* literally 'image-making'. Prinzhorn wasn't interested in querying the aesthetic worth of these images because he saw every single image made by people, even unconsciously made scribbles and doodles, as expressions of a human mind. So might these images open up a road to other minds? Prinzhorn, for one, claimed that 'all expressive gestures as such are subordinate to one purpose: to actualize the psyche and thereby to build a bridge from the self to others' (p. 13).[2]

Prinzhorn was not the first to come up with such ideas; in fact he was heavily influenced by the German philosopher Ludwig Klages, who had laid out his theory of expression in the book *Ausdrucksbewegung und Gestaltungskraft* (roughly: *Movement of Expression and Creative Force*), first published in 1913 and referenced to by Prinzhorn in the second edition of his text (1921). Following Klages, Prinzhorn interprets expressions as 'materialisation of the soul' (p. 12).[2] The English translation refers to the 'capability of realizing psychic elements' in 'expressive gestures' (p. 12).[2] However, the German original is 'Ausdrucksbewegungen haben die Eigenart, Seelisches zu verkörpern', which, firstly, explicitly mentions the soul and, secondly, sees expressions as 'embodiments'. He sees images as 'expressive facts' (*Ausdruckstatsachen*) and he additionally assumes that there is a biological drive in humans to create and thereby to express themselves (p. 13).[2] Hence, everybody is expressing their inner world constantly in images and other products of creativity. The 2006 exhibition of 'outsider art' at the Whitechapel Gallery in London was therefore aptly entitled, *Inner Worlds Outside.*

Prinzhorn also introduces a 'schema of the tendencies of configuration' (p. 14), which might be read as a template for his claims about the normal functions as well as pathologies of expression (p. 12).[2] Klages developed the idea of an urge for expression in yet a different direction and laid the groundwork for graphology, the analysis of handwriting, which supposedly enables inferences about people's personality. Yet this expansion of the approach is probably more of an example of its pitfalls.

The general idea, though, to see efforts of the creative mind as messages from the elusive realm of the subjective standpoint, was popular at the time. Other philosophers and art theorists were developing similar theories in the early years of the twentieth century. Leo Tolstoy, in his essay 'What is Art?' had already written in 1896:

> Speech, transmitting the thoughts and experiences of men, serves as a means of union among them, and art acts in a similar manner. The peculiarity of this latter means of intercourse, distinguishing it from intercourse by means of words, consists in this, that whereas by words a man transmits his thoughts to another, by means of art he transmits his feelings.[3]

Hence works of art, according to Tolstoy, are means to access an aspect of the inner world of others, specifically their feelings. In the same vein, Robin G Collingwood later described works of art as a kind of language in *The Principles of Art* (1938). And even today, in a textbook on the philosophy of art, one can find similar statements, for instance: 'Art provides the evidence of things not seen' (p. 263).[4]

Images, in contrast to their source (the human mind) can be directly experienced. Hence, the paintings that Prinzhorn collected might be used as a means to access the minds of mentally ill people, if only indirectly. But even if we agree with the general outline of the theory of expression, we might still wonder what exactly we might be able to learn from studying those images. How closely are the mind and its creative products linked? How much of a truthful mirror of subjectivity are these images? And, more importantly, how can we be sure that they are represented in our, the perceiver's, mind, in an undistorted way? After all, it takes another subjective mind to interpret the message from the other's mind.

Prinzhorn was well aware of these problems. In order to address the latter one, he again referred to a contemporary philosopher, this time Edmund Husserl, who had introduced the notion of *Wesensschau* (intuition of essence). The idea was that in order to get access to other minds the receiver or contemplator had to be in a certain frame of mind, which lets him understand the message intuitively – a kind of empathy. Obviously, with his own background in psychiatry and art history, Prinzhorn was supposedly well equipped to understand the mentally disordered mind of psychiatric patients.

This was not a scientific methodology he proposed. In fact, it was explicitly contrasted with a scientific perspective, which aims at causal explanations of the mind and mental disorder (p. 273).[2] However, these restrictions need not pose limitations, as it all depends on the purpose of the exercise. Prinzhorn focused on using his study as a means to understanding expressions of troubled minds, hence to get a better grasp of what it is like to suffer from schizophrenia. He didn't want to use his findings as a tool of diagnosis: 'We cannot say with certainty that any given picture comes from a mentally ill person just because it bears certain traits' (p. 265).[2] Finally, Prinzhorn was at pains not to infer too much from the studies of his samples; all his findings were regarded as hypotheses.

The other methodological problem, which has to do with the potential lack of authenticity of pieces of art, might arguably be less severe in the particular area of psychiatric artistry. Patients usually don't have a conscious plan for their creative outputs, in contrast to many professional artists. Their works might therefore more truly be authentic expressions of their minds. Still, one needs to proceed carefully here: some information about the context in which particular pieces had been made was also required. For instance, were they commissioned, possibly with a particular task in mind? Or were they produced simply because patients felt the urge to express themselves?

THE MAIN CHARACTERISTICS OF PSYCHIATRIC IMAGES

Prinzhorn made an attempt to derive general descriptions of some of the features he identified in the images of his collection. This effort aimed to lead to a grasp of the patient's worldview. Again, in terms of methodology it needs to be said that the identified general elements of psychiatric images did not stem from the perception of empirical evidence but were based on the 'intuitive experience' (*Erschauen*) of the contemplator – Prinzhorn himself.

There are four primary characteristics or peculiarities of schizophrenic configuration that are introduced in Prinzhorn's book. They are not necessary nor altogether sufficient criteria of 'insane art', but general features, which might be found in images made by psychiatric patients and which can give evidence of their state of mind. This is not proof that their state of mind is pathological; I have already emphasised that Prinzhorn did not want to use his findings for diagnostic purposes.

Firstly, Prinzhorn identifies a dominance of playful elements and an uninhibited urge to decorate, lacking in any overarching formal order in some of the samples. Contrary to many professional pieces of art, these images are not laid out according to a particular plan, but seem to follow a stream of consciousness. In terms of a formal aspect of images, they lack in coherence and consistency. One of the examples, a drawing by Barbara Suckfüll illustrates these elements (*see* Plate 3). It is a mix of words, written in neat handwriting, and kitchen utensils, with contours made of numbers. There is no unifying scale – spoons, cups, etc. come in unrealistic proportions – nor is there a fixed viewpoint, as all the words are arranged in different angles.

Secondly, Prinzhorn refers to a peculiar feature he calls 'ordering tendencies'. He mentions the lack, or at least mere sketchiness, of a plan or ordering motive. He also claims that there is sometimes a kind of pointlessness, insofar as, for instance, shapes are iterated without resulting in a meaningful composition. The example provided here (*see* Plate 4) is a painting by August Klett, which Prinzhorn dubs 'playful-decorative paper'. It is a colourful expression, containing shapes and ornamental elements, but also representational components like faces and animals. There does not seem to be a point which this image might be aiming at.

The third element Prinzhorn describes is a divergence of representational features (the way something is pictured) and regulatory features (the order of expression). This can occasionally be seen in a vehement drawing style, which undermines possible representational intentions; a lack of rhythm, as it were. The example reproduced here (*see* Plate 5), painted by Hermann Beehle, manifests a related divergence. It supposedly shows a sacral figure or idol. The figure is mostly made of geometric shapes. For Prinzhorn, this points at a discrepancy between the tendency to actually represent something, in this particular case a figure, and the way of expression, which in this case dwells on ornamental scribbling.

The fourth peculiarity of schizophrenic imaging is concerned with the content, in contrast to the aforementioned formal elements. Prinzhorn identifies a preference for ambiguous, enigmatic and mystic content and a lack of focus on the real world. He also believes that this artistic preference usually relates to subjectively significant themes, especially religious, erotic and magic elements. In the impressive painting by Franz Karl Bühler (*see* Plate 6), we see 'The Exterminating Angel', obviously a personification of anxieties, which also bears religious connotations. Admittedly, Bühler's case is special, as he was a trained artist and was therefore better equipped to represent in his paintings a specific world-view than laypersons.

Having identified a number of characteristics of the image-making of psychiatric patients, Prinzhorn attempts to establish an interpretation or understanding of what it is like to be mentally ill, or to experience schizophrenia, to be more precise. He believes that a common feature is a feeling of alienation from the world and other human beings, something he calls autism. Interestingly, he also uses the term 'solipsism', which I have introduced above. Schizophrenic art, according to Prinzhorn, shows signs of autistic separation from the world, which can culminate in solipsism, that is, the feeling of being alone in the world. As we have seen, images made by people who feel estranged from the world and fellow human beings in this respect might function as messages which can be used to get in touch with, and bring back to a common world, persons whose mind is somehow disturbed. The study of those images might therefore be a valuable contribution to therapeutic efforts.

QUESTIONS AND PROBLEMS

This chapter is partly a plea to take seriously and develop Prinzhorn's efforts to use images by psychiatric patients to gain a better understanding of their situation and frame of mind. I have also said, on the other hand, that there are many pitfalls and unsolved problems surrounding this approach. In this section, I want to raise some questions and potential problems more explicitly and discuss how these may be used in an educational context.

Firstly, can we really infer the state of mind of individuals from single specimens of artwork? Prinzhorn used a huge number of images and he eventually drew quite general conclusions about the 'schizophrenic worldview'. But can we use a similar approach to find out about the point of view of single persons? After all, we often want to understand a particular person; we want to gain access to a single mind. There might be features, of course, which are common to all people experiencing mental illness, but that alone seems a steep claim. So what use might the study of particular paintings be if we focus more narrowly on an understanding of individual patients?

One possible solution to this problem might be to use more samples from a particular person. Surely we cannot understand the way a person thinks or feels from seeing one image he or she has made; but neither can we know a person well from talking to them only once. This is a common feature of getting acquainted with a person; it has no greater acuteness in psychiatry. If we have access to more artworks, we might be able, for instance, to study the particular style of a painter. Style seems to be a feature, after all, which points at a regular characteristic of a creator, barring inauthentic expressions, of course.

The proviso just mentioned points at another problem: the potential lack of authenticity. Is the meaning, for instance, that we see in an image the same meaning, if any, which the artist attached to it? Maybe the feeling of alienation is merely 'read into' the work of people suffering from schizophrenia. I have already addressed this problem briefly and suggested that patients usually don't follow an artistic or even financial purpose, which makes their work more likely to be authentic. It seems safe to assume that in unprofessional settings an artist expresses his or her feelings by painting without 'feigning'. However, there is one issue which hasn't been mentioned thus far. When Prinzhorn gathered the images and other works from all over Europe, there were no psychotropic drugs to alter the state of mind of patients. This suggests that there was a higher likelihood of 'seeing' messages from a disordered mind at that time in history. Today, it might be necessary to introduce methodological tools to account for the 'filtering', if you will, of mental outputs by psychiatric medication.

The final point concerns the frame of mind of the person who contemplates and interprets the images. In general, Prinzhorn's methodology requires considerable empathy and intuition from the contemplator and it may be queried whether this capacity is common in psychiatrists or other mental healthcare professionals. In fact, it might be considered a dangerous approach in that it can transfer to third persons a certain power of expertise about the mind of a patient. However, as long as we don't impose any such 'mind-reading' of patients on them, the communicative tool of image making might still be valuable.

CONCLUSION

Art has been used as a way to understand the mind of other people generally and to gain access to the 'disordered mind' in particular. Hans Prinzhorn's collection and his theory of the artistry of those with mental illness, combined with his more general account of the process of expression, is an especially remarkable example of such a pursuit. There are other examples one might like to mention, for instance

Leo Navratil's more recent studies about the relation of art and poetry to schizophrenia.[5] Navratil was the founder of a community of mentally ill artists in Gugging, near Vienna, which is now a thriving source for marketable outsider art. There is also a book by the Swiss psychiatrist Walter Morgenthaler, a contemporary of Prinzhorn's, about a particular patient artist, Adolf Wölfli, possibly one of the best-known outsider artists.[6] Interestingly, Prinzhorn's colleague at Heidelberg, Karl Jaspers, author of the celebrated *General Psychopathology*, also published studies on art and psychiatry in the year 1922; he was concerned with 'pathographies' of Strindberg and van Gogh.[7] There remains a wealth of material to be studied, not only in terms of scholarly work, but also in terms of art collections. For instance, Dumfries' Crichton Royal Institution in Scotland has even older samples than the Prinzhorn collection and most of it is fairly unknown.

Prinzhorn concluded that patients with schizophrenia suffer from an involuntary alienation from their environment, in contrast to the conscious alienation of the expressionist avant-garde artists of the time, whose work bears some similarities to psychiatric art. Further to his claims about the patients whose work he studied, he made a valuable attempt to develop tools which might help us understand patients. These valuable and interesting insights notwithstanding, his methodology and therefore his conclusions are certainly contestable. However, they should not be dismissed but developed and improved. Mental health professionals can gain much by studying psychiatric art.

SOME SUGGESTED TEACHING TASKS AND QUESTIONS

Note: It is important to help students understand that the suggested way of making inferences about other people's minds, particularly patients' feelings and viewpoints, is a potentially dangerous one. It is mainly a philosophical idea, although an interesting one, which might serve therapeutic benefits. It might also be worth trying to use this chapter as a starting point for a debate on the role of art therapy as described in Chapter 8, which is a different, but possibly related, idea.

➤ Explore the Prinzhorn Collection website. Look at some of the examples of artwork and try to identify any of the characteristics that Prinzhorn mentioned. www.prinzhorn.uni-hd.de/index_eng.shtml

➤ Read or listen to the interview with outsider artist Anthony Mannix and art theorist Colin Rhodes. Can you identify any parallels between outsider art and the artistry of the mentally ill? www.abc.net.au/rn/allinthemind/stories/2006/1586067.htm

➤ Can you think of different ways to access other people's minds? How do psychiatrists and mental health nurses do this in practice?

➤ Do you believe that creative products can express the state of mind of the creator? How would you argue in favour of your point of view?

➤ How can we make sense of the difference between explaining a disorder and understanding a patient? Is a scientific perspective ever sufficient, especially if we have a therapeutic aim?

➤ In what ways does a modern psychiatric hospital environment undermine the purposes of understanding patients through art?

BOX 4.1 Other useful resources

Collingwood RG. *The Principles of Art.* Oxford: Oxford University Press; 1958 (first edition 1938).

Fuchs T, Jádi I, Brandt-Claussen B, *et al.* (editors). *Wahn Welt Bild: Die Sammlung Prinzhorn.* Berlin, Heidelberg, New York: Springer; 2002.

Hayward Gallery (editor). *Beyond Reason: Art and Psychosis: works from the Prinzhorn Collection.* London: Hayward Gallery; 1996.

Heidelberger Kunstverein (editor). *Die Prinzhorn-Sammlung: Bilder, Skulpturen, Texte aus Psychiatrischen Anstalten (ca. 1890–1920).* Königstein: Athenäum Verlag; 1980.

Maizels J. *Raw Creation: outsider art and beyond.* London: Phaidon Press; 1996.

McGregor JM. *The Discovery of the Art of the Insane.* Princeton, NJ: Princeton University Press; 1989.

Rhodes C. *Outsider Art: spontaneous alternatives.* London: Thames & Hudson; 2000.

RöskeT. *Der Arzt als Künstler: Ästhetik und Psychoanalyse bei Hand Prinzhorn.* Bielefeld: Aisthesis; 1995.

TenigIF (Klages-Gesellschaft Marbach) (editor). *Klages, Prinzhorn und die Persönlichkeitspsychologie: Zur Weltsicht von Ludwig Klages.* Bonn: Bouvier; 1987.

Whitechapel Gallery (editor). *Inner World Outside.* London: Whitechapel Gallery; 2006.

Zolberg VL, Cherbo JM (editors). *Outsider Art: contesting boundaries in contemporary culture.* Cambridge: Cambridge University Press; 1997.

REFERENCES

1 Nettle D. *Strong Imagination: madness, creativity and human nature.* Oxford: Oxford University Press; 2001.

2 Prinzhorn H. *Artistry of the Mentally Ill: a contribution to the psychology and psychopathology of configuration.* Berlin, Heidelberg, New York: Springer; 1972.

3 Tolstoy, L. *What is Art? What is Religion?* (translated by Aylmer Maude, V Tchertkoff, AC Fifield.) Rockfield, MD: Wildside Press LLC; [1898] 2008. p. 41.

4 Eldridge R. *An Introduction to the Philosophy of Art.* Cambridge: Cambridge University Press; 2003.

5 Navratil L. *Schizophrenie und Kunst.* München: Deutscher Taschenbuch Verlag; 1965.

6 Morgenthaler W. *Madness and Art: the life and works of Adolf Wölfli.* Lincoln, NE: University of Nebraska Press; 1992.

7 Jasper K. *Strindberg and van Gogh: an attempt of a pathographic analysis with reference to parallel cases of Swedenborg and Hölderlin.* Tucson, AZ: University of Arizona Press; 1977.

CHAPTER 5

Poetry and clinical humanities

Femi Oyebode

INTRODUCTION

Paul Valèry wrote that '[Poetry] is the attempt to represent, or to restore, by means of articulated language those things, or that thing, which cries, tears, caresses, kisses, sighs, etc.' (p. 147).[1] Valèry is here remarking on the especially close relationship between the passions and poetry, signalling the way in which poetry is a ready source of how we respond to distress, how we negotiate crises, and in what ways language can be used to obscure, disclose, disguise or dissemble feeling.

In this chapter, I will examine: a) the use of poetry by poets who have experienced emotional disturbance; and b) the writings of doctor-poets. Both categories of writings provide examples to illustrate the varying roles of literature in clinical education; giving accounts of the lives of sick people and their stories, and describing the lives of clinicians and the difficulties inherent in their roles.[2]

There is at present little literature on the use of poetry in clinical teaching. There is no published material on what poems might be useful and how these poems might be used. This is not to say that the place of poetry in the teaching of clinical humanities is limited in scope or peculiarly problematic, but to remark on the paucity of published material on the subject. This, despite the fact that poetry ought to have a privileged position: poems are often short and can be read at one sitting, and may also be read aloud and analysed as a joint activity within a teaching session.

The aims of the medical humanities as set out by the Association for Medical Humanities include: a) to emphasise education as distinct from training; b) to contribute to the development of students' and practitioners' abilities to listen, interpret and communicate, and to encourage their sensitive appreciation of the ethical dimensions of practice; c) to stimulate and encourage a fitting and enduring sense of wonder at embodied human nature; and d) to develop students' and practitioners' skills in thinking critically and reflectively about their experience and knowledge.[3] These aims can be met by the use of poetry in clinical teaching. Since poems are not directly about clinical skills, they help to emphasise the importance of a broader education, an awareness of the rich cultural resources available to clinicians and patients alike, underpinning our common humanity. The skills required to read, comprehend and fully decode a poem are the same skills required for active listening in a clinic: apprehension of the multilayered content of language and its infinite capacity both to express and to obscure. Poetry by its nature calls attention to alternative perspectives, challenges a simple biomechanical understanding of the world, and inevitably reflects and explores the perilous fragility of the human condition.

It is unarguable that the clinician's role is both to be technically competent as well as humane in his approach. Being humane involves connecting and engaging with the patient's concerns and worries, the patient's understandings as well as misunderstandings, and drawing from the same pool of cultural motifs as the patient, so as to grasp the patient's apprehensions. Literature, and poetry by extension, provides a ready source, an insight in to what Scott calls 'the common and shared patterns of response to critical situations, or into unique and individual responses to crises',[4] and may also enrich the language and thought of the clinician.

Our clinical, technical language can and does set us apart from patients. At the time when the patient is most in need of support and understanding, clinical language can create a wider gulf, thereby isolating the patient from our proper concern. John Diamond described it thus: 'When things go wrong we find ourselves hostage to men and women who use language we don't understand, talk of scientific principles we don't have the learning to grasp, who seem to be more confident than their results would allow, who offer us treatments which seem to work on some random basis which is never explained to us' (p. 31).[5] What literature can do is to give access to a fund of notions and experiences not incorporated in clinical texts. Poetry can also give clinicians access to the language in which distress is mediated, expressed or controlled. This process is not appreciated enough; poetry and literature give all of us the language to express the inexpressible or the common experience that is unique when it happens to us. In practice, this means that clinicians can engage with patients using a common language to discuss the human dimension of clinical dilemmas.

POETRY OF DISQUIET
Materials
The poems of Elizabeth Jennings (1926–2001), Robert Lowell (1917–77), John Burnside (b. 1955), Ivor Gurney (1890–1937), Stevie Smith (1902–71), Anne Sexton (1928–74), John Berryman (1914–72), and John Clare (1793–1864) are good sources of material that deal with emotional distress and its manifestations, consequences and clinical management.

1. Administering madness
Elizabeth Jennings' poems, 'A Mental Hospital Sitting Room', 'Sequence in Hospital' and 'Night Sister' deal with the theme of the hospital environment, the waiting rooms and wards, and the patience of nurses.[6] The poem 'Visitors' by Robert Lowell

deals with how mental health legislation is administered by describing the intrusion by two policemen into his home to detain and remove him to hospital.[7] The poem 'The Asylum Dance' by John Burnside deals with one of the many rituals of the nineteenth-century asylum, the annual dance.[8]

These poems all illustrate aspects of the patient's experience of what it is like to receive care within the mental health system. Except for the poem by John Burnside, they are written from the patient's perspective and draw attention, as only poetry can, to minute, almost negligible details, in order to emphasise or to make fresh our comprehension of the particular situations under scrutiny. An example of this is Lowell's description of the policemen as 'fat beyond the call of duty', hereby hinting at the excesses of power and coercion in the process of detention and removal.

2. Melancholia

The poems by Ivor Gurney, 'To God', 'The Shame', and 'An Appeal to Death' are expressive of anguish, emotional pain, despair and the wish for death.[9] They are direct and speak to us from a place of utter darkness. Stevie Smith, in 'Not Waving but Drowning', 'The Hostage' and 'Come Death' also speaks from a desolate place but the language is whimsical, quirky and comical by turn.[10] This allows for the student to see the varying registers in which anguish can be declaimed.

The poem 'Eleven Addresses to the Lord' by John Berryman[11] and Elizabeth Jennings' 'Michelangelo's Sonnets'[6] are in the form of prayers and demonstrate how despair can be communicated through prayer thereby highlighting the desperation implicit in despair. Finally, John Clare's, 'I Am' is an example of the poetic voice still aspiring to life and self-esteem even in the throes of despondency.[12]

JEALOUS MISTRESS

Materials

There is a tradition of doctor-writers that includes such illustrious authors as Arthur Conan Doyle, John Keats, Oliver Goldsmith and others. Anton Chekhov (1860–1904) memorably described the tensions inherent in the task of being both a practising doctor and writer: 'Medicine is my lawful wedded wife and literature is my mistress. When I get tired of one I spend the night with the other'.[13] It is unclear why anyone writes, or why doctors in particular write, but it is likely that there are aspects of clinical practice that simulate what is required for writing: the capacity for observation of physical mannerisms or abnormalities; for careful recording of social interactions; and participation in human tragedy or positive, uplifting events as an actor in the events. The writings of doctors, particularly their poetry where it deals with medical practice are worthy of study. These poems by doctor-poets often illustrate: the aims of medicine; nostalgia for what has been lost in modern medical practice; the impact or the strain of medicine on doctors; and the insights about life and death from the vantage point of medicine. There are poems by Charles Ingraham (1852–1935), James Matthews (1853–1910), Spencer Free (1856–1938), Dannie Abse (b. 1923), Glenn Colquhoun (b. 1964), Vincent Hanlon, Kirsten Emmott,

Elmer Abear, Ron Charach (b. 1951), Lenrie Peters (b. 1932), and William Carlos Williams (1883–1963).

1. Nostalgia

Ingraham's 'Frightening Death', Matthews' 'A Ballade for Busy Doctors' and Free's 'The Old-time Family Doctor', are poems that look back to a time when doctoring did not necessarily aim to cure (because treatments were ineffectual or unavailable), but yet medicine provided care and comfort.[14,15,16] These poems serve as a reminder that technological advances can and often do undermine the caring aspect of clinical care. Dannie Abse's poem 'In the Theatre' describes neurosurgery in the early part of the twentieth century and reveals the arcane art of medicine that both sets doctors apart and privileges their knowledge of the human body.[17]

2. Compassion fatigue

Glenn Colquhoun's poem 'Today I Do Not Want to be a Doctor', is an example of how a clinician might respond to the apparently unending burden of caring for others.[18] The poems by Hanlon ('A Lover's Quarrel'), Emmott ('Junkie on the Phone' and 'A Memorable Story') hint at the cynicism that can undermine compassion within the clinical context.[19,20] These poems exemplify the difficulty in retaining empathy and compassion and provide the basis for discussion about the risk of detachment and callousness on the one hand and of undue emotional enmeshment and compassion fatigue on the other.

3. Life and death

Abear's poem 'House Call' and Charach's 'A Poem About the Pancreas', are poetic responses to clinical situations, namely of forlorn old age and of the lethality of carcinoma of the pancreas, respectively.[21,22] Peters' 'Watching Someone Die' and Williams' 'Complaint' deal with the polar opposites of death and birth.[23,24] These poems exemplify what Ulla-Carin Lindquist meant when she wrote 'To work as a doctor is a privilege, with all the contact it gives, all the insights into life, dying and death'.[25]

ACTIVITIES

1. Small group teaching

It is best to work in small groups of 10–12 students. The learning objectives should be explicit and include: a) privileging language; b) understanding the roles of literature in clinical education; c) understanding the emotional life of sick people; and d) why clinicians write and what they write about.

The texts to be used should be available in advance of the sessions so that students can prepare for the session by reading and reflecting on the content of the poems.

2. Reading out loud

It can be helpful for students to take it in turn to read the relevant poems out loud.

The teacher can model this by starting the group off and getting the students to volunteer as the session progresses. There is something about poetry that enriches the sessions by the act of reading aloud. The best poems are written for the human voice.

3. Interpretations
The students should be encouraged to contribute to the sessions with their own understanding and perspectives on the poems. This teaches the students that alternative interpretations are equally valid, that interpretations are tentative, and that literary texts are open to fresh meaning. The sessions gain in value if they are supported by real examples from clinical practice or from the life experience of the participants. Thus, the poems should serve as the basis of a discussion that points outwards, aiming at subjective, individual or collective experiences of the participants.

4. Link to other literary texts
It is useful for the students to see how poetry relates to other literary texts. This can be accomplished by drawing the students' attention to how the themes exemplified by the poems are handled in fiction, autobiography, letters or journals. The poems that deal with melancholia can be complemented by readings from books such as William Styron's *Darkness Visible* or Tim Lott's *The Scent of Dried Roses*.[26,27] In much the same way, the poems on life and death can be further elaborated by Ulla-Carin Lindquist's *Rowing Without Oars* (25) or John Diamond's *C: because cowards get cancer too* . . .[25,28]

ASSESSMENTS
Essays are probably the best assessment method for clinical humanities courses, coupled with presentations to the group. The essays should be of 2000–3000 words, written to a title such as 'Critically discuss with references the role of poetry in medical education' or 'Discuss the statement: 'Poems by doctor-poets potentially undermine clinical detachment and objectivity'. The students should have the opportunity to summarise their essay in a 15-minute presentation to their peers and to respond to questions and comments from colleagues.

CONCLUSIONS
This chapter has drawn attention to a wide range of poets and their writings, including poets who are recognised as having experienced psychiatric disorders and doctor-poets who have a special, more intimate relationship with the subject matter of clinical practice. What is clear by any reading of these sources is the intensity of the literary material and the directness with which these poems deal and trade in distress and anguish. Students in all clinical professions are exposed to human distress and anguish on a daily basis, and poetry is a safe and illuminating way to explore and deal with the feelings and thoughts that accompany these experiences.

RESOURCES

Barritt P. *Humanity in Healthcare: the heart and soul and medicine.* Oxford: Radcliffe Publishing; 2005.

Oyebode F (editor). *Mindreadings: literature and psychiatry.* London: RCPsych Publications; 2009.

www.lannan.org The Lannan Foundation is a family foundation dedicated to cultural freedom, diversity and creativity. It has an audio archive of recordings of major writers including poets.

www.poetryarchive.org This is the leading online collection of recordings of poets reading their works.

www.poets.org This is a project of the Academy of American Poets. The website has poems, poet biographies, essays, interviews and poetry recordings.

REFERENCES

1 Valèry P. *Selected Writings of Paul Valèry.* New York: New Directions Publishing Corporation; 1950.

2 Charon R, Trautmann Banks J, Connelly JE, *et al.* Literature and medicine: contributions to clinical practice. *Ann Intern Med.* 1995; **122**: 599–606.

3 Arnott R, Bolton G, Evans M, *et al.* Proposal for an academic association for medical humanities. *J Med Ethics: MH.* 2001; **27**: 104–5.

4 Scott PA. The relationship between the arts and medicine. *J Med Ethics.* 2000; **26**: 3–8.

5 Diamond J. *Snake Oil and Other Preoccupations.* London: Vintage; 2001.

6 Jennings E. *New Collected Poems.* Manchester: Carcanet Press; 2002.

7 Lowell R. *Day by Day.* New York: Farrar Strauss and Giroux; 1975.

8 Burnside J. *Selected Poems.* London: Jonathan Cape; 2006.

9 Gurney I. *Collected Poems.* Kavanagh PJ (editor). Manchester: Carcanet Press; 1982.

10 Smith S. *Selected Poems.* London: Penguin Books; 1975.

11 Berryman J. *Collected Poems 1937–1971.* London: Faber and Faber; 1989.

12 Clare J. *Selected Poems.* Bate J (editor). New York: Farrar, Strauss and Giroux LLC; 2003.

13 Chekhov A. Letter to Alexei Suvorin, 11 September 1888. In: Hellman L (editor). *The Selected Letters of Anton Chekhov* (translated by S Lederer). Hopewell, NY: The Ecco Press; 1994. p. 54.

14 Ingraham CA. Frightening death. In: McDonough ML (editor). *Poet Physicians: an anthology of medical poetry written by physicians.* New York: Granger Book Co. Inc; 1945. p. 98.

15 Matthews JN. A ballade for busy doctors, op. cit. p. 100.

16 Free SM. The old-time family doctor, op. cit. p. 108.

17 Abse D. *Collected Poems 1948–1976.* London: Hutchinson; 1977.

18 Colquhoun G. *Playing God.* Auckland: Steele Roberts Ltd; 2002.

19 Hanlon V. A lover's quarrel. In: Charach R (editor). *The Naked Physician.* Ontario: Quarry Press; 1990. p. 51.

20 Emmott K. Junkie on the phone/A memorable story, op. cit. p. 65.

21 Abear E. House call, op. cit. p. 99.

22 Charach R. A poem about the pancreas, op. cit. p. 125.

23 Peters L. Watching someone die. In: Lowbury E (editor). *Apollo: an anthology of poems by doctor poets*. London: The Keynes Press; 1990. p. 149–50.

24 Williams CW. *The Collected Poems 1909–1939*. Manchester: Carcanet; 1987.

25 Lindquist U. *Rowing Without Oars* (translated by M Myers). London: John Murray Publishers; 2004.

26 Styron W. *Darkness Visible*. London: Jonathan Cape; 1990.

27 Lott T. *The Scent of Dried Roses*. London: Viking; 1996.

28 Diamond J. *C: because cowards get cancer too . . .* London: Vermillion; 1998.

CHAPTER 6

When art and medicine collide: using literature to teach psychiatry

Arun Chopra

INTRODUCTION

> When we read alone and for pleasure, our defences are down – and we
> hide nothing from the great characters of fiction. In our consulting rooms,
> and on the ward, we so often do our best to hide everything, beneath the
> white coat, or the avuncular bedside manner. So often, a professional
> detachment is all that is left after all those years inured to the foibles, fal-
> lacies and frictions of our patients' tragic lives. It is at the point where art
> and medicine collide, that doctors can re-attach themselves to the human
> race and re-feel those emotions which motivate or terrify our patients . . .
> Every contact with patients has an ethical and artistic dimension, as well
> as a technical one.[1]

AIMS OF THE CHAPTER

Duncan Macmillan House is an imposing Victorian building that was formerly an
asylum, at the edge of Nottingham city. Nowadays, with the city's enlargement, it
occupies a less peripheral position and is the headquarters of an NHS mental health
trust. It no longer serves as a hospital. Thoroughly modernised from the inside, it
still retains an impressive but somewhat sombre visage. Each time I enter, I wonder
what life was like for those who lived or were incarcerated there.

Much of this chapter was written sitting in the library of Duncan Macmillan
House, opposite a section devoted to 'fiction and mental illness'. Its shelves hold
a wide range of literary styles and works from Bronte's *Jane Eyre*, through F Scott
Fitzgerald's narrative of a troubled psychiatrist, *Tender is the Night*, to more recent

books like Mark Haddon's accurate portrayal of the world as experienced by a young man with autism, *The Curious Incident of the Dog in the Night Time*.

Six years ago when I started work as a junior doctor, this section of the library's catalogue didn't exist. Today, judging by the steady stream of visitors, it is one of the most used sections. What this large collection of books illustrates is how pervasive mental illness themes are within our culture and how rich a resource these fictional accounts are in the training and further development of mental health professionals.

Over the last few years, I have had the opportunity to teach psychiatry to both postgraduate and medical undergraduate students. Hesitantly at first, I started to use examples of characters from books and films to illustrate psychopathology, diagnoses and the complex psychosocial problems that often accompany mental illness. I thought that this approach might clarify and reinforce concepts that students often described as abstract. What could be more 'real' than the character suffering from morbid jealousy in *Enduring Love* (1997), who stabs the rival for his love in delusional rage?

Soon after they started, the 'literature' sessions were over-attended. Anyone who has ever tried to maintain the enthusiasm of students on late Friday afternoons will know, this was a considerable achievement.

A couple of years later, the opportunity to teach undergraduate medical students as part of a humanities-based module looking at the links between arts and psychiatry arose. Since then I have led the seminar on 'Literature and Psychiatry' as part of the module.

There is a growing awareness of the usefulness of medical humanities within the medical curriculum. However, the idea that this is an 'add-on' to the mainstream curriculum remains prevalent. Writing in 1999, at the introduction of a new journal on medical humanities, Evans and Greaves noted: 'In many ways, the position of the medical humanities resembles that of medical ethics 20 years ago, when its modern form emerged in Britain as an absorbing academic discourse but not yet the integral part of medical education and practice that it has now become'.[2]

The situation has improved since then, however the use of humanities is still viewed as a peripheral supporting activity rather than a mainstream method of imparting knowledge, skills and attitudes. When I started using these methods a few years ago, other clinicians would comment on how the students would appreciate doing 'something' a bit different and how they might gain 'something' from it. Although I appreciated their acceptance of my teaching style, implicit in their comments was the notion that at best, the humanities would just add 'something' and were not an integral factor in medical education. Richard Smith has observed: 'The additive view is that medicine can be 'softened' by exposing its practitioners to the humanities; the integrated view is more ambitious aiming to shape the nature, goals and knowledge base itself'.[3]

I am aware that some people are sceptical about the approach that this chapter, and indeed this book, takes and they believe that the arts are too 'woolly' to impart meaningful knowledge to the student. There are commentators who suggest that the arts do not make people more sensitive. Harold Bloom, a literary critic, has observed that reading literature is a selfish activity and does not necessarily make us better, more caring people; it can expand our intellectual horizons but does not engender a sense of altruism.[4] Oscar Wilde famously declared that 'All art is quite useless' and denied any suggestion that it could be educationally or morally uplifting. After considering both the pros and cons of reading literature, Beveridge concludes that it is up to the individual psychiatrist to decide whether literature is worth exploring in his or her professional development.[5]

This chapter is a practical guide to establish a session using literature to teach psychiatry. I will also consider the arguments in favour of using literature to teach psychiatry as this might be discussed at such a session. The chapter also includes a list of resources that could be used, however these are not explored at any great length. Oyebode has provided an excellent account of many of the resources that could be used.[6]

WHY USE LITERATURE?

Theoretically, using literature as a method of teaching psychiatry is aligned to two approaches to learning: experiential[7] and constructivist.[8]

Heron defined experiential learning as 'knowledge by acquaintance' in literal or symbolic form and involving action, reflection, emotion and imagination.[6]

Literature is a form of experiential learning that involves symbolic experience and appeals naturally to the learner's imagination. It elicits an emotional response from the reader as they identify with characters' joys, struggles and aspirations.

Constructivism fosters learning by encouraging the discovery of meanings through the use of personal viewpoints and validation of the learning experiences through intersubjectivity or the convergence of personal meanings.[7] Literature as a teaching tool presents opportunities for both personalised and intersubjective learning. Experiential learning and constructivism share the assumption that true learning is rooted in evocative learning. Unlike with the largely cognitive-oriented traditional didactic teaching, experiential or constructivist based learning methods appeal to emotions and provoke thought, and therefore achieve a higher learner level of retention long after the initial learning episode.[6,9]

Often, health issues are presented to students in a decontextualised manner, which can detract from student interest and learning. Fictional accounts can contextualise the symptoms and articulate the experience of suffering in a memorable manner. Further, literary works engage the reader more fully by engaging their imaginative faculties. In literary accounts, portrayals of suffering can go beyond the terms of nosological classification. This makes the description of the illness more vivid. For example, in *Darkness Visible: a memoir of madness*, William Styron rejects the very term 'depression' as an inadequate word for the suffering he has been through.[10] He describes it as 'a true wimp of a word for such a major illness'.

Understanding the patient and carer experience

Patient narratives are a key source of information about the experience of receiving care. Understanding this experience helps professionals in providing care tailored to patient need and in developing empathy. There is a paucity of information about the patient experience, other than from academic journals or textbooks, although increasingly the Internet is proving to be a source of patient narratives, for example www.healthtalkonline.org. Although surveys presented in research papers are useful sources in conveying the difficulties that patients face, they do not describe the emotions and difficulties that patients and their carers go through. The clinical records can be difficult to access and often contain only the facts and interpretations by professionals. Recently, there has been an effort to encourage patients to add their 'narrative' to the clinical record. However, the uptake has been low. At the time of acute illness, many patients might not be able or wish to contribute a narrative to their record, and on recovery, with the multiple teams involved, there is a lack of clear locus about whom should request such a narrative and where it is best held.

Currently, fiction provides a useful way through which professionals and students can tap into the subjective experience of the patient. As Oyebode has observed:

> What the arts and humanities can do for psychiatry is to reinforce the importance of the subjective. Our current diagnostic approaches emphasise the objectivity of symptoms and understate the importance of how these symptoms are experienced by people; this despite the fact that the roots of clinical psychopathology lie in phenomenology.[11]

Understanding psychopathology

Some texts can provide good examples of psychopathology. The worked example in a later section of this chapter illustrates this. Although there is no substitute for bedside clinical teaching with real patients, literature can provide a method of consolidating knowledge about psychopathology.

Awareness of the self

A work of literature is perceived in different ways according to our differing interests, personalities and varied life experiences. It is inevitable that our past experiences shape the understanding of the text that we are reading. How then, can we use a literary text to aid students' understanding of psychiatry when each student will perceive the piece of work somewhat differently? Rather than limit the use of literature, the varied responses actually illustrate a useful learning point that can be applied to the understanding of psychiatric practice. ICD 10 diagnostic classification not withstanding, we each approach patients differently, and more clearly remember or relate to different aspects of their stories. And by discussing these differences in interpretation we can understand more about our roles within the treatment dyad.

Literature can facilitate self-reflection. Works such as Camus' *The Plague* and Chekhov's 'Ward No. 6' delve into the personal, professional and political lives of a doctor and a psychiatrist. The following excerpt from 'Ward No. 6' illustrates the difficulties faced by a professional:

> Having looked the hospital over, [Dr] Ragin concluded that it was an immoral institution, detrimental to its inmates' health in the ultimate degree. The wisest course would be to discharge the patients and close the place down, he felt, but he decided he lacked the willpower to accomplish this on his own . . . Having taken the job, Ragin adopted an attitude of apparent indifference to the irregularities . . . Ragin much admires intellect and integrity but lacks the character and confidence to create a decent, intelligent environment.[12]

Therapeutic reading and relaxation

Careers within the healthcare profession are rewarding but they are also stressful. Developing the practice of reading for pleasure can be one way to deal with stress. As Sir Aubrey Lewis advocated:

> [The medical doctor] must have not only vocation, but avocation, some-thing which will call him further away into other fresher fields than those of his daily work. Such an avocation is literature . . . It teaches him to see his own work in its right perspective, not divorced from other forms of knowledge to which it is complementary nor sundered from other arts with which it is united.[13]

Reflective practice

Medical students are expected to maintain portfolios with documentary evidence of achievements and competencies. Students often find it difficult to produce reflective pieces. This might be because of the lack of reflection time they have given the intensity of the medical curriculum. In addition, medical students might struggle with the actual process of reflecting on their feelings. After the 'arts in psychiatry' module we conducted interviews with students. They reported 'surprise' when they were asked how they 'felt' about a patient. They suggested that medical school had taught them to value facts far above feelings. Medical humanities might help them develop reflective skills and find a medium through which they might express themselves.

Developing skills in medical ethics

Literature provides an interesting approach to exploring moral dilemmas. William Carlos Williams, a doctor and a writer, presented in a short story 'The Use of Force' (1938) the dilemma of whether force is ever justified in a medical intervention. Although the situation in this story is a young girl's reluctance to allow the doctor to examine her throat, mental health professionals are often confronted with similar dilemmas about whether treatment should be imposed against a patient's will. Short stories have been used as a method of introducing psychiatric ethics to postgraduate residents.[14]

WHAT DO THE STUDENTS THINK ABOUT THIS APPROACH TO LEARNING PSYCHIATRY?

The use of literature to teach psychopathology has been well received by graduate students. Mpofu and Feist-Price reported that in response to open-ended questions about their experience with literature-based learning, the majority of graduate students reported that they remembered a greater number of the diagnostic features for schizophrenia much more readily following this learning than was the case with previous (undergraduate) learning when they deliberately committed these to memory using a variety of mnemonic devices.[15] Many also reported that stories provide contextual understanding and encourage critical thinking. All the students noted that they found the literature-based learning more engaging than the traditional didactic method.

In another study using short stories, Rudin, *et al.* reported that residents rated a literature and ethics seminar highly, as it increased their ethical sensitivity and they found the content of the stories stimulating.[14]

In our own experience we have found that students responded well to the session on literature. All students reported that they enjoyed the session and all felt that it would be useful to their future careers. In the research we conducted (Tischler, *et al.*), some suggested that being a medical student could be limiting in terms of self-development and having time to explore outside interests as the following quote illustrates:

> I certainly stopped reading fiction when I came to medical school and I think it is just 'cause the text books take over (David, male).[16]

HOW TO USE LITERATURE

Setting aims for the session

Sharing clear aims with students provides a framework that guides the session. A discussion of why literature has been used to deliver the specific educational aims of the session should be included. It might be that literature is only one way of many that could have been used; acknowledging this promotes student engagement. Whilst the educational aim ought to be clear at the outset of the session, the reasons for using literature as the means of delivery might be discussed at the end of the session. Having a clear educational aim helps to guide selection of text. For example, I wanted to use a piece of literature to illustrate the psychopathology of schizophrenia and therefore I chose Gogol's *Diary of a Madman* (1834), *see* Box 6.1.

BOX 6.1 *Diary of a Madman*: example of a précis and pre-session questions

I have used Nikolai Gogol's *Diary of a Madman* in several teaching sessions in order to illustrate the psychopathology of mania and teach the diagnostic concepts of schizophrenia, schizo-affective disorder and bipolar disorder.

I have included the précis that is provided to students ahead of the session along with suggested questions.

Diary of a Madman: introductory notes and suggestions for discussion

Gogol's *Diary of a Madman* is the story of the descent into madness of Axenty Ivanov, a low-ranking official in the Russian bureaucracy. It is set in the 1830s and is written in the form of a series of diary entries that demonstrate the increasing disintegration of the protagonist's mind.

Author

Gogol was born in 1809. He started to write plays and short stories whilst at school. He was determined to make his name as a writer and after leaving school he headed for the city of St Petersburg. The *Diary of a Madman* appeared in 1834. His most celebrated book, *The Overcoat*, was published in 1842. He wrote several other books and plays and achieved success as a writer. In his latter years he was afflicted with religious mania and despair. He died in 1852 after subjecting himself to a severe regime of fasting.

Possible areas for discussion

1. What evidence for illness does the diary contain? Can it be described in terms of the 'symptoms' and 'signs' of mental illness that we use today?
2. The protagonist seems to be looking forward to his journey to the hospital because he thinks that he is going to the Spanish Court. The patients we see differ in their levels of insight. Consider a modern-day patient developing a psychotic illness with little insight and sectioned under the Mental Health Act: How might they experience the journey to the hospital? How would they consider the treatment and the ward? How have things improved since Gogol's time?
3. In a *BMJ* paper, Althschuler (2001) argues that the story represents one of the oldest cases of schizophrenia. He suggests that it is a brilliant sketch of the illness. Why do we see so few reports about the illness from that period and before? (The discussion might include notions of illness and labelling, social functioning and schizophrenia, how societies deal with deviant behaviour, what makes a diagnosis and what are the benefits and drawbacks of a diagnosis in modern times).
4. What part of the story captured your attention, if any? Why?

Reference

Altschuler E. One of the oldest cases of schizophrenia. *BMJ*. 2001; **323**: 1475–7. Available at: www.bmj.com/cgi/content/full/323/7327/1475 (accessed 15 May 2010).

Selection of the text

The selection of text depends upon the facilitator's knowledge of literature as well as knowledge of the subject. There are many lists of books that are available from a variety of different resources that illustrate which text could be used for teaching a particular area. In this chapter, we include a suggestive list (*see* Table 6.1). Using a precompiled list to identify appropriate texts is a relatively easy way of finding suitable material, however, I would recommend discovering in one's own reading texts that might illustrate an aspect of psychiatry that would fulfill a useful learning objective.

It is worthwhile considering the emotional impact a particular text might have. Also, consider the author of the text. Topics such as the author's mental state at the time of writing the book, or the author's own experience of mental illness (if known) often stimulate discussions around the link between mental illness and creativity.

At first I found choosing an appropriate text a rather daunting challenge and I chose from pre-prepared lists. However with time, it became a reflexive skill and I would realise whilst reading a book that it would be a useful work to communicate an aspect of psychiatric practice.

TABLE 6.1 Examples of literary works that can be used in teaching

Title (year of first publication)	Author	Areas illustrated
The Long Way Out (1937)	F Scott Fitzgerald	Schizophrenia, ethics
The Plague (1947)	Albert Camus	Professional ethics
Ward No. 6 and Other Stories (1892)	Anton Chekhov	Psychiatric ethics
Diary of a Madman (1834)	Nikolai Gogol	Psychosis, mania
The Curious Incident of the Dog in the Night Time (2003)	Mark Haddon	Autistic spectrum disorder
The Bell Jar (1963)	Sylvia Plath	Depression, ECT
Enduring Love (1997)	Ian McEwan	Morbid jealousy
One Flew Over the Cuckoo's Nest (1962)	Ken Kesey	Institutional care
'The Use of Force' (1938)	William Carlos Williams	Ethics of care
Tender is the Night (1933)	F Scott Fitzgerald	Professional ethics
Asylum (1996)	Patrick McGrath	Nature and consequences of jealousy
Spider (1990)	Patrick McGrath	Psychosis
Human Traces (2005)	Sebastian Faulks	History of psychiatry
Jane Eyre (1847)	Charlotte Brontë	Stigma
Darkness Visible: a memoir of madness (1990)	William Stryon	Depression
Shame (1983)	Salman Rushdie	Intellectual Disability

It can be better to use less popular books. There is a risk in using the 'obvious' pieces, as time is always a scarce commodity and some students will have read the book and won't bother re-reading it. Others will think that they have a general sense of what happened in the book. Try to avoid using books that have been made into movies. The movie, which is the producer's vision of the book, soon becomes the 'gold-standard' view and other viewpoints unfortunately get drowned out. As I mentioned before, I once used *Enduring Love* to illustrate morbid jealousy. I asked the class to look through the book and identify evidence for the delusional beliefs of the unwell character, however, astonishingly it soon became clear that the only pieces of evidence that students managed to pick up on were the ones that Rhys Ifans portrayed in the film of the book.

I have tried using both short excerpts from a few books as well as whole books. In my experience, the latter works better. There is a temptation to use a few excerpts from multiple sources (in order to cover more areas), however in practice this is difficult. In order to have an informed discussion having more of the story rather than multiple excerpts is better. The only occasion where I have found multiple excerpts to be useful is where the sole educational aim was to illustrate psychopathology.

The length of the chosen text depends upon the time available before and during the teaching session. If the book is too long, then there is a difficulty in identifying key passages and much time is wasted during teaching with students flipping between the relevant pages and refamiliarising themselves with the issue under consideration. Tightly written shorter books with examples of speech or thought, work well. Short stories, though not as popular as novels in the literary world, work well for this style of learning. Writing about the use of literary classics in teaching medical ethics to physicians, Radwany and Adelson warn that short stories may not develop plot and characters as well as a play or a novel.[17] However, Rudin, *et al.*, who used short stories in teaching psychiatric ethics, found that a highly crafted, condensed short story provided extraordinary impact, emotional resonance, and ethical ambiguity.[14]

Background preparation and the start of a session

A good way to enhance student engagement is to distribute a précis of the piece with a brief summary of the author's biography. An example that we have used in our teaching is provided (*see* Box 6.1).

Questions that follow discussions on works of literature such as 'how did that piece make you feel?' are not commonly encountered in the medical curriculum and students often feel embarrassed to answer such questions. As students have pointed out, they are used to questions of fact and not to questions of feeling. Laying down ground rules to ensure confidentiality and respect for others' views helps to allay anxiety and allows for a more free discussion. Identify a contact person for students if there are problems that arise post-session.

Promoting engagement

As well as clear aims it is important to have clear tasks. The task should enable the student to meet the educational aim. I usually include primary tasks that are based on a reading of the text and secondary tasks that extrapolate from the text in order to facilitate a discussion around application.

Examples of the processes involved in establishing tasks follow:

1. Students often don't consider the experience of patients who are admitted to a mental health ward despite shadowing the junior doctor whilst they interview and examine the new patient. Unfortunately, due to time constraints and the necessity of objectivity, most admission notes report signs and symptoms but contain little of the 'experience' of the patient.

   In order to address this gap in understanding, I set the aim of a session – to consider the experience of becoming a patient. For this task I asked students to read an excerpt from Sylvia Plath's *The Bell Jar* and then: a) consider the emotions that are conveyed; and b) consider what similarities and differences they noted between Sylvia Plath's account of an admission and an admission in a modern day ward.

2. Electro Convulsive Therapy (ECT) is considered a stigmatising treatment and the general public perception of it remains negative, despite the fact that for some patients it can be life-saving. The aim set for the session was to consider the perceptions of ECT against the reality of treatment. I used the portrayal of ECT from the book, *One Flew Over The Cuckoo's Nest*, as the session's text. The tasks set were to: a) identify the similarities and differences between ECT as depicted in the book and the ECT they had observed; and b) consider how they would discuss the treatment with relatives and carers of a patient who was due to have ECT who had seen the film or read the book.

Different students will engage with the materials and tasks in different ways. It is also important to be aware that some students will accept this approach more readily than others. It can be quite a cultural change to be asked questions for which there are no right or wrong answers. For example, all students will answer a question on the first-rank symptoms of schizophrenia in approximately the same way. However, asking about the emotions that students pick up from a work of literature might lead to a variety of different responses and sometimes these will conflict. In my experience, where students have elected to take up a humanities module, they show greater willingness to engage in this approach and accept differences in opinion. However, in non self-selected groups, there can be a section of students who feel that this approach is 'wishy-washy' and 'not scientific enough'. It is that section of students who need to be reminded why this is a reasoned approach to educational aims if humanities-based modules are ever to be mainstreamed in medical education.

Organising responses

The task of the facilitator is to pick up on responses and use them to stimulate further discussion. This can be quite simple, such as thanking a student for volunteering their interpretation and then asking the group for their response. However, it can be difficult to develop any meaning from a number of varied responses to open-ended questions. Without developing some structure for students to place the information, opportunities for learning might be missed.

   Using a visual aid to record responses helps to prevent this. After eliciting responses these can be grouped together to aid retention. The visual record also acts as a prompt to stimulate further reflections. Occasionally, the group will provide responses that could not have been anticipated. It is important to be flexible so that opportunities to develop interesting ideas are available.

Whilst arts-based teaching is less formal than traditional didactic teaching, occasionally it becomes necessary to intervene and remind students of the original aims. In one memorable session we used excerpts from the book *Touched by Fire* by Kay Redfield Jamison to discuss links between mania and creativity. The conversation veered to hearing voices as a sign of manic psychosis. A student made a link between religious prophets and mental illness. The discussion continued for a short while, however as this was leading on to uncomfortable territory for some students, I intervened to bring the group back to the session aims.

Facilitating discussion and popular areas for discussion

Discussion flows from the responses to the tasks that have been set, however certain areas that form recurrent themes are:

➤ psychopathology: using actual examples of psychopathology and teasing out what this might mean in terms of a diagnosis

➤ psychosocial issues: the complexities of how and where care is provided and the ways in which families cope with mental illness

➤ medication: this often receives quite a negative depiction in literature and this is something that facilitators should be aware of. There are many reasons why this might be the case: perhaps those who write of their experiences are those who are not suffering from the more extreme forms of illness for which medication appears most useful, or perhaps medication is not as beneficial as the profession perceives it to be.

Application of the session to the 'real world'

The end of the session relates the discussion and what has been learnt to the real world, guided by the aims of the session. To consider one of the examples described above, at the end of our discussion on admissions to mental health wards, we agreed that patients might feel 'bewildered' on their first admission. However, there was also a realisation that many doctors don't acknowledge this when clerking in new patients. It was agreed that students would discuss with nursing staff how they approached the task of reducing the anxieties of new patients. Students felt that the session had impressed upon them the significance of acknowledging the distress that patients might feel on admission and the importance of multi-disciplinary teams.

Providing the opportunity for feedback

Provide the students with an opportunity to give feedback on the session. We have found it useful to gather both qualitative as well as survey-based quantitative data.

Costs and copyright

The sessions are not materially expensive. Costs to be considered are printing if you are planning to distribute copies of the text and teaching costs for any external speakers.

We used PDFs of the relevant pages that we were able to e-mail to the students taking the module. We also ensured that the books considered were available at the university libraries. Another consideration is copyright rules. Wherever there is any doubt it is useful to speak with the university legal service and/or the publisher.

RECRUITMENT CRISIS IN PSYCHIATRY

I was encouraged that students taking the humanities module I teach have expressed interest in pursuing a career in psychiatry. This is of particular importance currently as psychiatry is suffering from a shortage of trainees.[18]

CONCLUSION

I hope that this chapter has demonstrated the role that literature has to play in psychiatric education and has provided a framework to those keen to make use of it.

REFERENCES

1　Collier JAB, Longmore JM, Hodgetts TJ. Fame, fortune, medicine and art. In: *Oxford Handbook of Clinical Specialties*. 4th ed. Oxford: Oxford University Press; 1995. p. 413.

2　Evans M, Greaves D. Exploring the medical humanities. *BMJ*. 1999; **319**: 1216.

3　Smith R. Editor's choice: struggling towards coherence. *BMJ*. 1999; **319**.

4　Bloom H. *How to Read and Why*. London: Fourth Estate; 2000.

5　Beveridge A. The benefits of reading literature. In: Oyebode F (editor). *Mindreadings, Literature and Psychiatry*. London: RCPSYCH; 2009.

6　Oyebode F. Fictional narrative and psychiatry. *Ad Psychiatr Treat*. 2004; **10**: 140–5.

7　Heron J. *Group Facilitation: theories and models for practice*. London: Kogan Press; 1993.

8　Gadamer HG. *Truth and Method*. New York: Pantheon; 1975.

9　Knowles MS, Holton EF, Swanson RA. *The Adult Learner*. Houston, TX: Gulf Publishing Co; 1998.

10　Styron W. *Darkness Visible: a memoir of madness*. New York: Random House; 1990.

11　Oyebode F. Editorial: literature and psychiatry. *Ad Psychiatr Treat*. 2001; **8**: 397–98.

12　Chekhov AP. *Ward No. 6 and Other Stories, 1892–1895*. London: Penguin; 2002.

13　Lewis A. *Monograph Supplement 10*. Cambridge: Cambridge University Press; 1986.

14　Rudin E, Edelson R, Servis M. Literature as an introduction to psychiatric ethics. *Acad Psychiatry*. 1998; **22**: 41–6.

15　Mpofu E, Feist-Price S. Use of literature in teaching psychopathology: some strategies for health educators. *Academic Exchange Quarterly*. 2002; **6**(3): 49–55.

16　Tischler V, Chopra A, Nixon N, *et al*. Loss and tomorrow's doctors: student perceptions of the value of humanities teaching (under review).

17　Radwany SM, Adelson BH. The use of literary classics in teaching medical ethics to physicians. *JAMA*. 1987; **257**: 1629–31.

18　Channel 4 News. Psychiatry's UK recruitment crisis. 4 June 2009. Available at: www. channel4.com/news/article.jsp?id=3190557 (accessed 16 February 2010).

CHAPTER 7

Creative writing as reflective practice in health professions education

Emily Ferrara and David Hatem

INTRODUCTION

In the words of W Somerset Maugham, a physician-writer who tended the sick in London slums in the early twentieth century, 'the doctor . . . sees human nature bare'.[1]

Whether physician, nurse or therapist, the role of caregiver affords a sacred proximity to the undeniable mysteries of human existence: the trials of illness, the resilience of the human spirit and ultimate mortality of the body. The use of creative writing in health professions education has the potential to illuminate both the plight and might of caring for the sick. When harnessed as a tool to support reflective practice, creative writing's power goes beyond inspired story-telling to support the development of self-aware, empathic, humanistic practitioners who are poised to deliver quality patient care.[2]

RATIONALE/LITERATURE REVIEW

Reflection in medical education is defined by Sandars as 'a metacognitive process that occurs before, during and after situations with the purpose of developing greater understanding of both the self and the situation so that future encounters with the situation are informed from previous encounters'.[3] Creative writing as reflective practice is grounded in the literature and medicine movement which took hold as an established scholarly field more than 30 years ago. It is widely accepted that 'Literature and Medicine share a fundamental concern – the human condition',[4] and that both literature and medicine as fields of study have the capacity to promote 'depth of insight, acuity of perception, and skills in communication'.[5] Reflective practice and transformational learning pedagogy took wing in the 1990s, and most recently, the fields of narrative-based medicine[6] and narrative medicine[7] have emerged as conceptual frameworks for guiding the provision of effective and deeply humane care. Rita Charon promotes the 'centrality and privilege of story-telling' in clinical practice, asserting that narrative engages a continuum of 'attention, representation and affiliation'.[8] According to Charon, reflective writing serves as a seminal act of the representation aspect of this narrative continuum, an essential component of the process:

> Better than just talking about these things in a support group or venting session, the actual writing endows the reflections with form so that others can join the writer in beholding it . . . If they can capture it with greater force and accuracy, it means that they are perceiving it better as it occurs.[9]

The uses of narrative in health professions training – whether through applying narrative-based skills in the patient encounter;[10,11] journaling in response to critical incidents;[12] or writing parallel charts, that is, writing in ordinary language about the trainee's experience of the patient encounter[13] – are not uncommon. However, curricula employing narrative methods are often voluntary or elective in nature. In cases where narrative skills are a formal part of the required curriculum, these narrative components may be experienced by learners as a kind of 'window-dressing' rather than as an integral framework for the teaching of clinical skills. Making maximal use of narrative methods, including employing the humanities as an integral aspect of medical education, is argued to be a critical component in current efforts to enhance professionalism and humanistic development in medical trainees.[14]

The inclusion of narrative methods incorporating 'creative writing' as a form of reflective practice is even more scarcely documented in the medical literature, although there are a smattering of articles focused exclusively on the subject of poetry and other forms of creative writing used in medical education contexts, both at the medical student and resident learner levels.[15-21] Enhancing empathy and self-awareness, and increasing learners' appreciation of the perspectives of others (e.g. patients, peers) are common outcomes of these interventions. The writing of poetry by medical students 'appears to be one way students can make emotional sense of the different relational systems they encounter over the course of training', including their interactions with patients and their family members, and their relationships with various members of the healthcare team.[22]

The recognition of the honored tradition of physician-authors of the twentieth century, such as W Somerset Maugham, William Carlos Williams and Anton Chekhov is ubiquitous, as is the burgeoning number of contemporary literary works of poetry, essays, short stories and memoir written by physicians, nurses and other healthcare professionals. These can be found in many venues: from the popular press (*New York Times*) to leading professional journals (*Journal of the American Medical Association, BMJ*), to academic and mainstream publishing houses. There are a wide array of columns in health professions journals devoted to the reflective and creative output of physicians, nurses and therapists, as well as literary journals devoted to the illness experience. Two such premier literary journals created just within the past decade are: *Bellevue Literary Review*, based out of the Department of Medicine at NYU Langone Medical Center, New York City; and *ARS MEDICA: A Journal of Medicine, The Arts and Humanities*, based out of the Department of Psychiatry at Mount Sinai Hospital, Toronto, Canada. Both journals provide companion teaching tools to encourage utilisation of the readings in the context of health professions education. This broad overview of the state of medical-themed literature affirms the fact that being a doctor, nurse, or therapist (or being 'in training' to become one) can be transformational in nature. These stories of transformation appear to be of mythic importance to the culture as a whole, and to the ongoing development of the healthcare professions.

Thus, there is a need for formalised opportunities for active reflection and introspection in health professions education at all levels, in order to engage in a meaningful way with the sacred and meaning-making dimensions of caregivers' work.[23,24] At the University of California, San Francisco, Rachel Naomi Remen's successful efforts to establish *The Healer's Art*, an elective course for medical students launched in 1993, broke new ground in this arena. In the academic year of 2006–07, the course was offered at more than 53 medical schools worldwide.[25] Offering a creative writing course which draws on narrative, reflective practice, and literature and medicine traditions, is another effective way to stimulate active reflection and introspection by students, particularly those who are drawn to creative expression through the written word.

The experience of 'seeing human nature bare' – whether in the medical student's first cut into the cadaver, or a nursing student's first encounter with an actively dying patient – can be a challenge to process while performing the necessary duties of their respective roles. The raw material confronting students during the training experience has the potential to be life-altering and uniquely impacts the formation of each student's personal and professional identity. These intense experiences, often referred to as critical incidents, require a 'container' to support students in their effort to traverse the soul-making work of becoming a doctor, nurse or therapist – or in educational vernacular: to achieve the competencies associated with professionalism. This requires integration of the newly acquired scientific knowledge base and clinical skills with the individual's personal identity, in order to develop a cohesive professional identity.

One of the most critical aspects of this important integrative work is the development of self-awareness in medical, nursing and therapist trainees. According to Kearney and colleagues: 'Self-awareness involves both a combination of self-knowledge and development of dual-awareness, a stance that permits the clinician to simultaneously attend to and monitor the needs of the patient, the work environment, and his or her own subjective experience'.[26] Kearney reports that empirical data supports the effectiveness of reflective writing as one of two methods found to enhance self-awareness (the other being mindfulness meditation).

The critical incident report (CIR) is a form of reflective writing that encourages students to identify an incident encountered in the course of medical training that has raised feelings of conflict or emotion that the student may experience as needing resolution. Although the writing in and of itself may be helpful to support reflective practice in students, CIRs have been found to provide greater value when used as a focus for group reflection.[27]

Encouraging students to write reflectively about conflicts and emotions requires the provision of a safe place within which to allow the raw material to emerge. The first step is providing safety within the writing process itself; parameters laid out in expressive writing research methodology as outlined by James Pennebaker can provide faculty with a basis for framing reflective writing exercises in such a way to allow students to delve into particular aspects of their experience only when they feel ready to do so.[28]

Creative writing courses – particularly those which engage creative writing as a form of reflective practice – provide the 'container' to allow for exploration and expression of the otherwise untapped, yet insistently emerging unconscious/sub-conscious thoughts and ideas. This makes them available to allow a greater degree of integration of biological, personal and interpersonal learning to occur during the training years. Exploration of issues usually not discussed and/or formally processed within the traditional medical school curriculum may be addressed in this way, as an antidote to the 'hidden curriculum'. This has been described by Hafferty as 'the commonly held understandings, customs, rituals, and taken for granted aspects of what goes on in the life space we call medical education.'[29] The hidden curriculum is a major influence on the learning environment, fully surrounding students in their day-to-day work, and involving interactions which may at times fall short of the ideal presented in the formal curriculum. Thus, the hidden curriculum can have a devastatingly negative effect on students' ability to maintain their sense of purpose and meaning in the face of the realities and limitations of clinical practice. It is hypothesised that the hidden curriculum contributes significantly to growing student cynicism as their training progresses,[30] indirectly teaching students to abandon idealism and their own personal identity and values to the detriment of their effectiveness, satisfaction and longevity in the profession.[31]

Shapiro, Kasman, and Shafer describe a model of reflective writing outlined as a linked continuum of writing, reading and listening. This process appears to be highly effective and practical in achieving pedagogical goals to enhance professional development, patient care, and practitioner well-being.[32]

WHAT WORKS WELL

Since 1998, University of Massachusetts Medical School (UMMS) has offered a creative writing elective to second-year medical students, as a mode of reflective practice – offering students an opportunity to reflect on the process of becoming a physician while in the midst of the most intensive delivery of medical information and required regurgitation – the passive form of learning typical of the 'preclinical' years of medical education. This elective has been found to serve three primary functions that support the development of students' professionalism competencies: 1) to enhance capacity for reflection and self-awareness; 2) to reduce stress and burnout; and 3) to bring attention to the spiritual aspect of the profession, supporting learners' determination to maintain connection with their own humanity, and reinforcing/ reinvigorating their original, humanistic reasons for entering the profession. The elective achieves this by providing a formalised curriculum in which to engage in reflection regarding the larger context of meaning and purpose in medicine.[33]

We offer students an opportunity to become active and reflective learners, defining, describing, and in some instances fantasising about the experiences of medical training during this early phase of indoctrination, into the professional code of values. This transformation is particularly striking in medicine in its breaking of taboos and crossing of boundaries not typically spanned by the average person: the dissection of the cadaver, the asking of personal questions and examination of intimate body parts as a standard practice of the profession. The creative writing elective provides an outlet for exploring these aspects of medical practice, including the expression of disillusionment with the realities of doctoring, the emotional toll of being in the presence of suffering, and the process of letting go of the person who entered medical school to that of becoming a physician – a transformation inherent in this type of professional training. These have emerged as 'narratives of resistance': the expression of narratives in opposition to the inevitable, the loss of control over one's life, the acceptance of the physician's role in society, and the experience of realising that mastery of medical knowledge is an unattainable goal.[34]

We have found that creative writing exercises grounded in reflective practice, and triggered by critical incidents serve as a useful method for surfacing and addressing difficult encounters, uncertainty, lack of clarity of role, feelings of inferiority, the strains of being at the bottom of a hierarchy, and the anticipation of future responsibility for the lives and well-being of patients.[35]

These are major tasks of professional identity development in medical students, and the creative writing elective provides a method and supportive environment for students seeking support for this aspect of their medical training experience. With critical incidents as a focal point, students are empowered to identify aspects of their experiences that have raised conflict or disturbing feelings in their medical training for potential resolution. In the context of this course, reflective writing about critical incidents enables our learners to identify challenges and discuss them more objectively, utilising the writing process and the creation of a story or poem to serve as a 'third thing' – providing a semblance of distance and objectivity to support the learner's ability to reflect meaningfully and non-judgmentally on these challenges.[36]

Further, the writing alone is not the endpoint; when followed by sharing and discussion of the writings as a part of the process, the benefits deepen. The construct of creating a community of fellow writers with whom to share drafts and receive feedback provides an opportunity to use the group as a 'sounding board', or simply as a witness to the student-writer's experience. As students are learning the importance of listening to patients in the context of their clinical training, the ability to listen deeply – to oneself, through the development of self-awareness, and to each other in the context of the sharing and feedback components of our creative writing course

– is a critical skill that translates into the students' work with patients at the bedside. Thus, the process of creative writing, and sharing this with others, has the potential to ultimately lead to better patient care.

The focus is on the writing 'process' versus the writing 'product'. The purpose of the course is not to complete finished works for publication, but rather to use the writing process creatively to reflect on the experience of 'becoming a physician' at a particular point in medical training, to share those experiences with a community of peers, and have the opportunity to give and receive feedback. Of note, we provide a resource listing of publishing opportunities for students interested in publishing their writing; in some cases, students have pursued publication, entered their work in writing contests, and created medical blogs. These are optional activities driven by students' level of interest; faculty make ourselves available to those students who are interested in furthering their writing, and publishing.

In our work with medical students during the past 12 years, we have identified the characteristics that have contributed to our ability to implement and sustain an effective creative writing elective for medical students. Based on our experience, we present several best practices to consider in developing and implementing a course of this type.

Homogeneity (in terms of year of study) of student participants

The homogeneity of the student participants was a positive feature of the experience: all were second-year medical students in their first semester of their second year of medical training; their career trajectory in medicine was still 'undifferentiated'. In terms of our particular medical school's curriculum, this meant that participants would have had a year's worth of required clinical experience interacting with patients through the Longitudinal Preceptor Program (LPP) and the Physical Diagnosis Course (PD). The LPP places students in the outpatient setting, in order to practise their skills in medical interviewing and physical examination, working under the supervision of a practicing physician. The Physical Diagnosis course provides students with the opportunity to gather medical histories and perform physical examinations on hospitalised inpatients who have given consent. Some students also avail themselves of other elective/enrichment opportunities, including volunteering in free clinic settings (established for patients who are uninsured), community-based patient screenings and summer immersion experiences in international clinic settings. The homogeneity of the medical student group drew on the students' shared experiences in the medical school curriculum, and capitalised on peer-to-peer engagement based on this shared experience. The value of the creative writing elective was intrinsic not only to the writing itself, but also to the opportunity to share perspectives and discuss the writing (both narrative form and content), to illuminate and broaden their own individual perspectives to global themes.

Length and format of course sessions

The Medical Creative Writing elective at UMass Medical School is designed as a seven-session course, conducted in the fall semester of each academic year. Each session is 1.25–1.5 hours in length. Due to the limited session length, and with the goal of being able to read aloud and provide in-class feedback on students' writings, the optimum maximum number of participants is eight students. Since this is an elective, the students who enroll come with the required element for creativity: self-motivation. Our goal is to provide them with the tools, the space and the community within which to explore their responses to the assignments, and to reflect on the transformational process of 'becoming a doctor'.

There is no text required for this course, in order to keep the students' focus on generating their own writings, and responding to each other's drafts. Students' writings in response to the assigned writing exercises serve as the 'text' for the course. Optional readings are provided – as samples of medical-themed creative writing.

Ground rules for sharing and feedback

In the first session, we set the stage for establishing a safe and confidential environment that will foster honesty, openness and bonding among the participants during this course. We discuss ground rules and guidelines, with a focus on creating an environment of confidentiality and privacy, and invite students to recommend additional parameters for group consideration. The faculty provides a framework for giving feedback on each other's writings. The framework for feedback is as follows: feedback is provided during the classroom session by both faculty and fellow students; students are invited to identify the type of feedback they are looking for to develop their piece of writing, e.g. they may request feedback on 'technical' aspects of the writing (clarity, use of language, point of view, tone) versus a general response to the 'story' or 'narrative'. We also offer students the opportunity to debrief the experience of reading their work out loud prior to inviting feedback from fellow students or faculty. It is important to note that reading the writing aloud to the group is optional; infrequently, we have had students decline to read, but the majority of participants share their writing during the sessions. One way that the faculty can establish a sense of trust within the group is to put themselves 'on the firing line' at the first session by reading a personal piece of writing of their own, and receiving feedback from students. This gives faculty a chance to model and students a chance to practise giving feedback to a less vulnerable member of the group. We have found that this strategy promotes equality and transparently communicates the intention of establishing a community of writers as a critical goal of the experience. Guidance for running sessions is given in Box 7.1.

BOX 7.1 Tips for running creative writing sessions

What works well:
- setting ground rules to ensure confidentiality, safety and respectful feedback; Faculty sharing own writing at kick-off session
- elective offering ensures participant motivation, promotes engagement
- offering a menu of writing topics grounded in critical incidents (*see* Box 7.2)
- providing for flexibility in terms of genre, length of assignments

- framing creative writing as a tool/method for reflective practice
- engaging students in peer-to-peer feedback, as well as offering faculty feedback.

What to avoid:
- dictating specific assignments
- devolving into grievance or gripe sessions
- setting out to be therapeutic (e.g. group therapy). Keep the focus of feedback on the writing itself, rather than the subject; discuss the subject, author, character as a way of allowing for some distance in discussion of the experience. Although our intent is not therapy many find the experience of the writing course cathartic and some find it therapeutic.

Assignment overview

The menu of writing topics is drawn from CIR literature. The topics are simple and wide ranging rather than being directive and proscribed. The first two assignments ask students to reflect on themselves and their own motivations, while the third assignment invites them to reach outside themselves to something that is considered 'known territory' – that of a student-teacher interaction (which can be from any point in their lives). The next two assignments focus on patient stories, placing the students' reflections squarely in the medical context. The final assignment – on balancing personal and professional life – is a challenging topic; we have found this to be most effectively addressed toward the end of the elective once a community of trust has formed, allowing students to write in a revelatory manner about their personal experiences and challenges. For suggested assignments *see* Box 7.2.

BOX 7.2 Suggested creative writing assignments

Session 1 *A Significant Experience in Medical School.* Write about a significant experience in medical school, whether positive, negative or mixed.

Session 2 *Becoming a Doctor.* Write about your decision to become a doctor, your experience as a medical student or your uncertainties about this process.

Session 3 *Memorable Student-Teacher Interaction.* Write about a memorable student-teacher interaction, whether positive, negative or mixed.

Session 4 *A Memorable Patient.* Write about a memorable patient you have encountered, whether the experience with this patient was positive, negative or mixed.

Session 5 *Voice: Memorable Patient from the Perspective of the Patient.* This can be a reworking of the Session 4 assignment, or a completely new piece of writing on a different patient.

Session 6 *Balancing Personal and Professional Life.* Write about the challenges you have experienced, or opportunities you have pursued, for balancing the personal and professional aspects of your life during medical school.

In response to all of the assignments, students are encouraged to draw from their own experiences, or the experiences of family members, friends or loved ones. Course participants may respond to the assignment prompts in any genre: narrative nonfiction, short story, poetry. There are no specific length restrictions or requirements. The assignments intentionally allow for a great degree of flexibility, enabling students to use the elective to write about and reflect on those issues identified as most important to them (assignments are open to interpretation by the students). Our intention is to counter the proscriptive and rote nature of much of the required curriculum in their first two years of medical school, and to prepare students for the broad range of positive and negative interactions that they will likely encounter in their clinical rotations during their third and fourth years of training. This may provide an opportunity for full and interactive engagement in a transformative learning model.

Although these assignments are focused on the medical student experience, these simple, straightforward assignments lend themselves to adaptation for use with medical students at a later stage of training, and with trainees in other health professions, including nursing, psychology and social work.

Offering this elective to second-year medical students comes at a particularly pivotal time in our students' development. Students may avail themselves of this opportunity to use the elective to explore uncertainties that may plague them early in medical training, particularly regarding the ubiquitous questions that most medical students had to respond to as part of their application process, questions that return to challenge their carefully crafted and well-considered essays and personal statements, once they are ensconced firmly yet seemingly precariously in their medical training: Why do I want to become a physician? Is this the right career path for me? What does it mean to be a physician? What are my options for a career in medicine? In the safety of the creative writing elective, students may choose to engage with the following questions: What will I have to give up to become a physician?, What am I gaining from the experience? What is the value of this experience? The opportunity to critically and creatively explore and respond to these developmentally appropriate questions, under new circumstances, can have great value to advance role and goal clarification, allow the self-assessment necessary for students to optimise learning about themselves, their patients and the medical profession, and to discern the best fit for choice of medical specialty.

Resources
Database
➤ **NYU Literature, Arts and Medicine database:** A resource rich in media that can provide inspiration and serve as a springboard for ideas in developing writing assignments and readings. Access is free of charge, and available through: http://litmed.med.nyu.edu/Main?action=new.

Medical-themed literary journals
➤ *Bellevue Literary Review*: This journal of humanity and human experience is published twice a year by the Department of Medicine at NYU Langone

Medical Center. For information, go to: http://blr.med.nyu.edu/
- ➤ *ARS MEDICA*: This journal of medicine, the arts and humanities is published twice a year by the University of Toronto Press. For information, go to: www.ars-medica.ca

Books on theory and practice database
- ➤ *Narrative Medicine: honoring the stories of illness* (Charon R). New York, NY: Oxford University Press; 2006.
- ➤ *The Therapeutic Uses of Creative Writing* (Bolton G). London: Jessica Kingsley Publishers; 1999.
- ➤ *Writing Works: a resource handbook for therapeutic writing workshops and activities* (Bolton G, Field V, Thompson K, editors). London: Jessica Kingsley Publishers; 2006.
- ➤ *Narrative-Based Medicine* (Greenhalgh T, Hurwitz B). London: BMJ Books; 1998.
- ➤ *Opening Up: the healing power of expressing emotions* (Pennebaker J). New York, NY: The Guilford Press; 1997.

Medical-themed literary works
These books are ideal for inspiration, and provide a storehouse of writing samples from a wide range of perspectives, including physicians, nurses, health professional trainees, patients and family members.
- ➤ *Between the Heartbeats: poetry and prose by nurses* (Davis C, Schaefer J, Trautmann Banks J, editors). Iowa City, IA: University of Iowa Press; 1995.
- ➤ *Intensive Care: more poetry and prose by nurses* (Davis C, Schaefer J, editors). Iowa City, IA: University of Iowa Press; 2003.
- ➤ *A Life in Medicine: a literary anthology* (Coles R, Testa R, editors). New York, NY: New Press; 2002.
- ➤ *Body Language: poems of the medical training experience* (Jain N, Coppock D, Brown Clark S, editors). Rochester, NY: BOA Editions, Ltd; 2006.
- ➤ *Kitchen Table Wisdom* (Remen, RN). New York, NY: Riverhead Trade 1997; 2006.
- ➤ *The Best of the Bellevue Literary Review* (Ofri D, editor). New York, NY: Bellevue Literary Press; 2008.
- ➤ *Ten Years of Medicine and the Arts: a hundred selections from academic medicine 1991–2001* (Dittrich LR, editor). Largo, MD: Association of American Medical Colleges; 2003.
- ➤ *On Doctoring: stories, poems, essays* (Reynolds R, Stone J, editors). New York, NY: Free Press; 2001. (All genres represented, includes many classics.)

REFERENCES
1 Maugham WS. The summing up. In: Donohoe MT. Perspectives of physician-authors of the past century on the practice of medicine. Manuscript Collection no. 56A.1.2, History & Special Collections for the Sciences, Louise M Darling Biomedical Library. Los Angeles: University of California; 1988.

2 Charon R. Narrative medicine: a model for empathy, reflection, profession, and trust. *JAMA*. 2001; **286**(15): 1897–902.

3 Sandars J. The use of reflection in medical education: AMEE Guide No. 44. *Med Teach*. 2009; **31**(8): 685–95.

4 Donohoe MT. Perspectives of physician-authors of the past century on the practice of medicine. Manuscript Collection no. 56A.1.2, History & Special Collections for the Sciences, Louise M Darling Biomedical Library. Los Angeles: University of California; 1988.

5 Churchill LR. Why literature and medicine? In: Donohoe MT. Perspectives of physician-authors of the past century on the practice of medicine. Manuscript Collection no. 56A.1.2, History & Special Collections for the Sciences, Louise M Darling Biomedical Library. Los Angeles: University of California; 1988.

6 Greenhalgh T, Hurwitz B. Narrative-based medicine: why study narrative? *BMJ*. 1999; **318**(7175): 48.

7 Charon R. *Narrative Medicine: honoring the stories of illness*. New York: Oxford University Press; 2006.

8 Charon R. Narrative medicine: attention, representation, affiliation. *Narrative*. 2005; **13**(3): 261–70.

9 Ibid.

10 Greenhalgh T, Hurwitz B. Narrative-based medicine: why study narrative? *BMJ*. 1999; **318**(7175): 48.

11 Launer J. New stories for old: narrative-based primary care in Great Britain. *Fam Systems Health*. 2006; **24**(3): 336–44.

12 Branch WT. Use of critical incident reports in medical education: a perspective. *J Gen Intern Med*. 2005; **20**(11): 1063–7.

13 Charon R. *Narrative Medicine: honoring stories of illness*. New York: Oxford University Press; 2006.

14 Shapiro J, Couhelan J, Wear D, *et al*. Medical humanities and their discontents: definitions, critiques, and implications. *Acad Med*. 2009; **84**(2): 192–8.

15 Bregman B, Irvine C. Subjectifying the patient: creative writing and the clinical encounter. *Fam Med*. 2004; **36**(6): 400–1.

16 Das Gupta S, Charon R. Personal illness narratives: using reflective writing to teach empathy. *Acad Med*. 2004; **79**(4): 351–6.

17 Hatem D, Ferrara E. Becoming a doctor: fostering humane caregivers through creative writing. *Patient Educ Counsel*. 2001; **45**(1): 13–22.

18 Kasman D. Doctor, are you listening? A writing and reflection workshop. *Fam Med*. 2004; **36**(8): 549–51.

19 Reisman AB, Hansen H, Rastegar A. The craft of writing: a physician-writer's workshop for resident physicians. *J Gen Intern Med*. 2006; **21**(10): 1109–11.

20 Shapiro J, Stein H. Poetic license: writing poetry as a way for medical students to examine their professional relational systems. *Fam Systems Health*. 2005; **23**(3): 278–92.

21 Shapiro J, Kasman D, Shafer A. Words and wards: a model of reflective writing and its uses in medical education. *J Med Humanity*. 2006; **27**: 231–44.

22 Shapiro J, Stein H. Poetic license: writing poetry as a way for medical students to examine

their professional relational systems. *Fam Systems Health.* 2005; **23**(3): 278–92.

23 Horowitz CR, Suchman AL, Branch WT Jr, *et al.* What do doctors find meaningful about their work? *Ann of Int Med.* 2003; **138**(9): 772–5.

24 Branch WT, Suchman A. Meaningful experiences in medicine. *Am J of Med.* 1990; **88**(1): 56–9.

25 ISHI programs and workshops: The healer's art: awakening the heart of medicine [course description]. Available at: www.commonweal.org/ishi/programs/healers_art.html (accessed 15 May 2010).

26 Kearney MK, Weininger RB, Vachon MLS, *et al.* Self-care of physicians caring for patients at the end of life. *JAMA.* 2009; **301**(11): 1155–64.

27 Branch WT, Suchman A. Meaningful experiences in medicine. *Am J of Med.* 1990; **88**(1): 56–9.

28 Pennebaker JW. Telling stories: the health benefits of narrative. *Lit Med.* Spring 2000; **19**(1): 3–18.

29 Hafferty FW. Beyond curriculum reform: confronting medicine's hidden curriculum. *Acad Med.* 1998; **73**(4): 403–7.

30 Haidet P, Dains JE, Paterniti DA, *et al.* Medical student attitudes toward the doctor-patient relationship. *Med Educ.* 2002; **36**(6): 568–74.

31 Krasner M, Epstein R, Beckman H, *et al.* Association of an educational program in mindful communication with burnout, empathy, and attitudes among primary care physicians. *JAMA.* 2009; **302**(12): 1284–93.

32 Shapiro J, Kasman D, Shafer A. Words and wards: a model of reflective writing and its uses in medical education. *J Med Humanity.* 2006; **27**: 231–44.

33 Ferrara E. The saving grace of vulnerability: fostering reflective practice in medical students through creative writing. In: Byers J, Forinash M. *Educators, Therapists and Artists on Reflective Practice.* New York, NY: Lesley/Lang Series Publishers; 2003.

34 Ibid.

35 Hatem D, Ferrara E. Becoming a doctor: fostering humane caregivers through creative writing. *Patient Educ Counsel.* 2001; **45**(1): 13–22.

36 Gaufberg E, Batalden M. The third thing in medical education. *Clin Teach.* 2007; **4**(2): 78–81.

CHAPTER 8

An introduction to art psychotherapy

Mariangela Demenaga and Daphne Jackson

INTRODUCTION

The British Association of Art Therapists (BAAT) defines the practice of art therapy as 'a form of psychotherapy that uses art media as its primary mode of communication'.[1] This means that the psychology of mark-making and symbolism are of intrinsic importance. The act of mark-making deepens the therapeutic understandings derived from psychotherapy alone, and empowers the client with a language beyond words. Practice may vary in accordance with client need, the context and the therapist, but the aim is to facilitate change by means of the potent activity of mark-making. This requires visual literacy as well as psychotherapeutic knowledge and skills in the therapist, who seeks to provide the necessary containment within the boundary of a therapeutic relationship.

In this chapter, we outline the theoretical basis of art therapy as an intervention stemming from human creativity and psychotherapeutic thinking, describe the process of art therapy and use case vignettes to illustrate clinical application of this form of therapy.

Since the 1940s, artists and art teachers have offered their services to hospitals and clinics, and psychiatrists and psychoanalysts have found drawings and paintings to be a valuable contribution to the therapeutic process. The profession of art therapy has developed considerably from this informal beginning, and training is now at postgraduate degree level.

'Art Therapist' and 'Art Psychotherapist' are both titles that are protected in law. Practitioners must gain their art psychotherapy qualification from an accredited institution and maintain registration with the Health Professions Council (HPC).[2] The HPC regulates the practice of Allied Health Professionals (AHP). Compliance with the HPC Code of Ethics and satisfying their requirements for continuing professional development (CPD) is essential.

THEORIES OF CREATIVITY

Links between art and therapy can be found throughout human history. A more formal approach and the development of art therapy as a profession is relatively new.

Rank examines the 'long and intricate path' that leads from the 'creative impulse' and envisions it as working 'directly in the service of [the] personality'.[3] May describes the creative courage needed to find 'new forms, new symbols, new patterns' as foundation for the future;[4] and Charles Stewart writes more specifically of the 'symbolic' process as a natural impetus that leads to maturation of the personality and psychological healing.[5]

The nature of art is 'one of the most elusive of the traditional problems of human culture', according to Wollheim.[6] It consistently resists definition, but prevails, occurring spontaneously throughout society. In the last century MacGregor celebrated the work of the clinically insane.[7] Dubuffet, himself an artist, collected it, as well as the work of 'those untouched by artistic culture' (l'Art Brut);[8] and Cardinal placed high value on 'creation springing directly from the original sources of emotion'.[9]

Perceptions of art and art movements have evolved throughout history, changing as the cultures from which they emerge have themselves evolved. Similarly, the range and use of media employed is limitless: naturally occurring pigments such as ochre precede materials that need deliberate and sometimes extensive preparation. Much forethought and preparation is required in the execution of a fresco, for example. To make a fresco, the artist needs a life-sized cartoon of the intended image which has been pricked out along the main lines, charcoal or other dust to blow through the pricked holes, and freshly mixed plaster and paint all ready before he/she can begin, because this must all be assembled on the surface before the plaster or paint dries. Before the modern era, the paint itself would also have to be freshly prepared by mixing pure pigment, which has itself been extracted from material such as ground vegetable matter, with a binding agent such as egg.

Art is a kinaesthetic activity in which the maker invests. It connects physical and mental, material and immaterial. Jackson Pollock said that 'Painting is a state of being . . . painting is self-discovery. Every good artist paints what he is'.[10]

Elkins, who dispenses with wavering distinctions between art and 'non-art', considers the expressive meanings of all images, referencing ongoing study of visual language in several fields.[11] Art in art therapy can be understood as a complex event within which process, product and context are all of significance. It permits exploration of created objects and the potential meanings granted to them.

The creation of images is ancient and universal. An art object survives from c. 70 000 BCE.[12] It comprises deliberate geometric marks, cut with a sharp stone tool, and may have symbolic purpose. Lewis-Williams in his study of the origins of art and the workings of the human mind, hypothesised that Upper Paleolithic art was shamanistic, thus linking the making of visual forms with religion and healing.[13]

When hunter-gatherers became farmers, mark-making further developed, diversified and became more articulate. Gimbutas notes a progressive increase in diversity over three millennia, such that more naturalistic expression was 'emancipated from an initial subordination to symbolic purpose'.[14] She convincingly extrapolates the cultural and religious import of Neolithic art and interprets forms that have their roots in Paleolithic art.

In the modern era, the 'ground paintings' of Australian Aboriginals are clearly religious rituals, and the sand paintings of the Navajo are sacred tools created by medicine men for the purpose of healing.[15,16] The order and symmetry of a painting symbolises the harmony that the subject wishes to re-establish in his or her life. Afterwards, the sand painting is considered to be toxic, since the illness is absorbed into it, and is destroyed. The art therapist works with the healing potential of the creative process, contained within the rituals of the therapeutic frame. Schaverien has made a study of this and her description of a 'successful picture' as one 'made up of conflicting elements which are held in resolution' implies something of the work.[17]

Calvino propounded that we live in a 'rainfall of images'.[18] An image is deceptively simple to see but can never be completely defined. Visually and viscerally, the impact is immediate, but on each review it can yield further meanings. The use of signs and symbols has been exploited for cultural, commercial and political purposes by means as diverse as flags, advertisements, statues and graffiti.[19]

Langer identified symbolisation as 'the essential act of mind' and specifically likened the brain to a 'great transformer' acting on the 'current of experience'.[20] Stevens supports this, stating that 'we possess an innate symbol-forming propensity which exists as a healthy, creative, and integral part of our total psychic equipment' and 'promotes our grasp on reality'.[21] Bachelard makes the point from the perspective of philosophy, describing a dialectics of imagination which 'would seize all that is real, and find more reality in what is hidden than what is visible'.[22]

Milner describes a process of reciprocity as making possible the symbolic expression of unconscious ideas so that art-making is a 'form of visual reflection on the basic problem of living'.[23] Rawson describes a process of search and consolidation, thoughtfulness and freedom. He sees rhythm at the root of all expression.[24] Art-making is kinaesthetic: lines may be cramped, expansive, and heavy, light, tentative, stabbed, scratched, swooping and swerving. Arnheim writes extensively on all aspects of visual perception, including colour and space.[25] Maclagan explores what he terms the 'facture' or particularities of the making; and Thomson gives many case examples of what is 'a form of human intelligence that is purely visual'.[26,27] Plate 7 shows emotions released into fluid media, chalk pastels and then paint.

The viewing or making of an image always introduces a personal factor. There is the prospect of narrative. Some kind of heterogeneous space occurs where the drama between seer and seen can be played out. Every art object bears the individual mark of its maker, conscious and unconscious. Personal imagery seems to have 'roots in a primordial pattern . . . enabling the individual psyche to preserve its unique form of expression at the same time as merging with the universally human'.[28]

The art product emerging from the process has a separate existence from its creator. It allows for communication and meaning but will be perceived by others in their own ways and according to their own experience and context.

PSYCHOTHERAPY THEORY

Art therapy draws from the vast literature on psychotherapy and its many approaches. Thinking as diverse as Freud, Jung, Bowlby, Lacan, Klein, Stern, Laing, Rogers and many others, may inform practice. A brief explanation of some key concepts follows.

Boundaries and containment

The establishment of containing boundaries is a prerequisite for the establishment of a therapeutic relationship, and vital in good therapeutic practice.[29] Essentially, it is this particular framing that makes the therapeutic experience distinct from other interactions.

The concept of the therapist as a container is rooted in the work of Bion. His concept of 'maternal reverie' refers to the state of mind of an infant's mother whereby she can (metaphorically) provide a digestive process for the infant's overwhelming feelings. This concept views the infant as projecting his/her intolerable, unshaped feelings of anxiety and dread onto the mother. She metabolises her infant's feelings and returns them in a form that can be accepted. However, if the mother fails in this process, the baby is left in a meaningless world of an obscure nature. Hinshelwood points out that Bion's concept of reverie is comparable with Winnicott's idea of holding.[30]

Winnicott describes the initial state of the dependant infant as a merging state with the mother/carer.[31] The baby born helpless to the world cannot be considered independently of the mother/carer or indeed survive if such a relationship doesn't exist. The quality of this relationship has mental and emotional bearing on the development of the infant. The good-enough mother is sufficiently attuned to the infant's emerging needs, creating an illusion of omnipotence for the infant (as if the external world is under the baby's magical control). In this, the mother creates an environment that embodies holding and containment. Thus, the environment is almost absolutely adapted to the infant. Gradually, attunement is lessened, disillusioning the baby and leaving him/her to slowly experience the frustration of reality where no omnipotent control is possible.

Along with the process of disillusionment, which can only take place if illusion exists in the first place, the baby moves from a state of absolute dependence to a state of relative dependence. So, to start with the good-enough mother – the person carrying out this process of illusion and disillusionment – acts as a container holding the infant. However, for the mother to be able to become engaged in such a way with the infant she needs to be held and contained herself in a supportive environment by a husband/partner, family, friends, the community, etc.

These concepts of Bion and Winnicott refer to the parent/infant relationship. Even if not used too literally in therapy, such analogies about the container and the contained help envision the therapeutic situation.[30] The client is held by and contained by the therapist within the therapeutic relationship through 'mirroring' and 'empathising'. In turn, the therapist, in order to provide such an environment, must be adequately held and contained in a supportive environment constituted by supervision, work environment, professional body, colleagues, networks, etc.

The therapeutic relationship

Searles, as quoted in Morter, argued that 'the therapist's face has a central role in this symbiotic interaction', thus helping the client to realise his/her 'own aliveness'.[32] He thought that facial expressions as a response to the client are analogous to those made by mothers responding to the baby. 'Empathic mirroring' further facilitates containment of the client by the therapist. This enables trust to develop and creates the function of the therapist as providing a supportive environment.

Bick conceives the infant as being in a state where personality and body parts are not yet differentiated from one another and are experienced as having no binding force among them.[33] An external object (i.e. the nipple in the infant's mouth) is experienced as able to hold together these otherwise unintegrated parts. The experience of these unintegrated parts being held together, when repeated over time, becomes introjected by the infant. Thus, the concept of an internal object, or what Bick calls a 'skin container', is formed. When this experience is reliably established, a sense of space inside the self can be created. This is central to being able to hold (own) and digest (process) experiences. If such space does not exist, the experience of emotion threatens the sense of self with annihilation. Similarly in therapy, tangible and psychological boundaries have the ability to hold and contain arising emotion. This draws further on the importance and relevance of boundaries and containment in the therapeutic setting. The person needs boundaries to frame a space within which to exist as an individual.

ART THERAPY

Art therapists are trained in art theory and psychotherapeutic thinking, as well as developing art therapy-specific theory. Art therapy was informed by Freud's work with dreams and free association, and also followed Jung's work with dreams, active imagination and archetypes. These make extensive use of visual imagery and are of primary relevance to art therapy.

In art therapy, the client's mental content is actively externalised through the art-making process. This sets off a tri-polar scheme of dimensions of communication, which are not mutually exclusive, but rather constantly interchangeable, succeeding and replacing one another. The dimensions of communication are shown in Table 8.1.

The therapeutic contract

The therapeutic setting, developed through the maintenance of boundaries will provide the client with the experience of a confidential space kept for him/her in each art therapy session.

The contract is agreed at the beginning of any art therapy intervention. It is a mutual agreement between the therapist and the client on the format and boundaries of the sessions. This will promote containment through consistency and create the foundations for a therapeutic alliance to develop from the beginning of the

TABLE 8.1 Luzzatto's dimensions of communication[34]

Expressive-Creative	Refers to client-image relationship.
	Provides client with a rich image making experience and is conducive to reaching symbolic imagery.
Cognitive-Symbolic	Refers to therapist-client relationship through the image.
	Aids the client in owning, sharing and understanding his/her work.
Interactive-Analytic	Refers to communication through the image in combination with direct therapist-client communication.
	The therapist offers him or herself as an object for the client's projections.

intervention. It will also allow the client and therapist to observe the boundaries and how they are used.

The client's expectations are discussed and information on this type of therapy is provided in an assessment interview. A number of assessment sessions will be agreed, which can take different formats (*see* Table 8.2), along with the boundaries. Following assessment, should client and therapist agree to continue, the contract (usually verbal) will be revisited and established. The components of the art therapy contract are seen in Table 8.3.

TABLE 8.2 Art therapy session formats

Individual	Therapist and client in one-on-one relationship.
Studio group	Group: art studio format where people are allocated an individual space and work in the presence of others. Membership may be open or closed.
Interactive group	People work individually or collectively on artwork and the focus is on interaction between members.

TABLE 8.3 Components of an art therapy contract

Time scale	Open ended or time limited.
Frequency	Usually one session per week. Day and time agreed and regular to reduce anxiety. Breaks are planned and responses to them talked about.
Venue	Must be consistent. Usually an art therapy room, if one exists.
Artwork	Kept safely by the therapist for the duration, usually in a personal folder. At the end the client may choose to keep or leave with therapist.
Non–directive stance of therapist	Client makes choices (themes, art materials, verbal interactions, use of time and space) for which he/she has responsibility and which can be reflected upon.
Reviews	Looking back at the body of work produced allows both client and therapist to reflect and gain new understandings on the work done and how it has evolved. This includes the use of media, emerging themes and the therapeutic relationship changing over time.

IMAGE-MAKING PROCESS

The use of art materials provide a tangible means via which conscious and unconscious aspects of the client's internal world can be expressed and brought to the outer world. Furthermore, this process can be observed in action and the resulting art product is physical and thus of actual and undeniable existence.

According to Winnicott, in normal development the infant becomes attached to a 'transitional object' (e.g. a dummy or blanket). This is instrumental in enabling the necessary shift from the earliest oral relationship with the mother to genuine object relationships.[31]

With the decathection of the transitional object, transitional phenomena 'become spread out over the whole intermediate territory between "inner psychic reality" and the "external world as it is perceived by two persons in common"' that is to say by the whole cultural field.'[31]

These phenomena are evident in play, artistic creativity and appreciation, religious feelings, dreaming and also fetishism, lying, stealing, origin and loss of affectional feeling, drug addiction and obsessional rituals.[31]

Play is a universal and healthy activity, facilitating growth and leading to group relationships. It is a form of communication. Winnicott argued that play has a time and a place that is neither inside nor outside the world of shared reality. He refers to this place and time as a 'potential space' and describes a third area of human living that belongs to the realm of 'transitional phenomena' – an intermediate area of experience. Being able to relax is a prerequisite to playfulness. The ability to play depends on creativity wherein the whole personality participates. In using the whole personality we have the opportunity to discover the self. In such a potential space the child plays alone in the presence of the mother, being witnessed and at times facilitated by her. In art therapy, when entering the therapeutic space, the client and therapist enter a safe space in which the client can relax. This depends on the containment provided by the boundaries that surround it. In Winnicott's words: 'psychotherapy is done in the overlap of two areas of play, that of the patient and that of the therapist'.[31] The creativity of the art therapist is thus a major therapeutic factor.

Through using art materials and reflecting on the resultant artwork in the presence of the therapist, the client has the opportunity to discover and to work with his/her own symbolism. Symbolism can reveal what is unconscious to what is conscious, thus creating a bridge. Symbolism consequently is of great value. Piaget, in his theory of cognitive development, considers that during the first sensorimotor stage from birth to 2 years of age, the infant develops the abilities of object permanence and of general symbolic function. In the latter, he distinguishes between the use of 'symbols' and 'signs'. Signs are conventional and have fixed meanings (e.g. words).[35] A symbol 'implies meaning greater than that that is immediately obvious'.[36] From a very early age people have the ability to represent symbolically. This is evident in the spontaneously emerging activity of mark-making in young children. The 'development from the basic scribble to the first representational drawings is a part of that development towards a semiotic or symbolic function, a development towards unique human consciousness'.[37]

INTRODUCING ART PSYCHOTHERAPY PRACTICE

Notwithstanding the rigorous thinking that underpins art psychotherapy, it is not an academic discipline. It is impossible to effectively convey the nature of what happens through words alone. It is essential to foster insight into the creative process, and to promote visual literacy.

Three major methods are proposed: (1) experiential learning; (2) reflection on the image; and (3) case studies.

Experiential learning

There is no substitute for physical engagement with art media and a workshop format is recommended. This enables participants to experience feelings, such as expectation, frustration, delight, excitement, fear and disappointment, which inevitably occur when one tries to find external form for internal experience. The specific foci of this type of learning in art therapy are included in Box 8.1.

BOX 8.1 Art therapy and experiential learning

- Qualities of different art media can be felt.
- Some materials are easier to control than others.
- Internal processes occur while working and can be observed.
- There is interplay between conscious intent and serendipity.
- Something made is unique, as is the hand that makes it.
- There is a relationship between maker and made.

It is important to note that self-reflection while making art invites unconscious processes and can quickly result in intolerable feelings of exposure. It can be extremely powerful and it is important that trained practitioners facilitate the process in order to protect from psychological harm.

Reflection on the image

Shared viewing of a piece of work promotes insight and the exchange of ideas. Individuals will see that the work is perceived differently in accordance with the culture and experience of each viewer. To view a famous artwork will encourage consideration of context. People can think together about all aspects of visual communication and discover some commonality in perception. For aspects worthy of consideration, *see* Table 8.4.

In art therapy, the process of reflecting with the client on his/her artwork is vital. In thinking about a vibrant red, for example, some may associate it with anger while others may associate it with love. In either case strong feeling is suggested and this fits with colour symbolism, as well as with the fact that, neurologically, red creates greater excitation than, for example, a soft blue.[39] However, the primary consideration is the meaning to the creator. The therapist's interpretation is never imposed.

TABLE 8.4 Aspects of image that are utilised in art therapy

Gesture	Weight of line
Direction of marks	Symbolisation
Small inflections of line	Use of picture plane
Colour	Narrative
Focus	Culture

During supervision the subjective experiences of the therapist are considered in the context of the work and its maker as well as the range of available theories.

Case studies

Two case vignettes are presented below. These encapsulate and effectively illustrate key elements of theories discussed in this chapter.

Vignette 1: My voices

Plate 8 was made by a 37-year-old male with a long history of reactive violence. The primary diagnosis was borderline personality disorder with associated psychotic aspects. The patient, whom I have named Jay, had a disturbed sense of self and was locked in routine and rituals to help him keep unwanted internal phenomena at bay. He was brought up within a strict God-fearing family where 'bad behaviour', including normal childhood 'naughtiness' was severely punished. For years he had heard voices: the voice of 'Thomas' (who had incited him to commit double murder) and the voice of 'Simon' who told him to 'chill'. Whilst formally accepting responsibility for his actions he did not really believe that a 'nice guy' like him had been the true perpetrator and was profoundly shocked that two people, both of whom he loved, had died at his hand. In his view 'Thomas' had committed the offences whilst he (Jay) was in a state of unknowing possession. He wished to be rid of the voices, but despite anti-psychotic medication, continued to hear them. On the whole he no longer acted on their commands and was a mostly compliant patient.

Jay presented as excessively verbal and controlled. He was anxious, joyless and judgemental, without capacity to play, and with an annihilating attitude towards his art. He could not use fluid media at first and all initial work was drawn in pencil on white A4 paper with a ruled containing margin. The image to be made was always chosen by him prior to his weekly session, outside the therapeutic frame, and was a tightly drawn construction, which was then explained to the therapist.

In Plate 8, Jay represents himself as a square, entirely separate from 'Thomas' who has 'sharp bits' and 'Simon' who is 'smooth' and with 'no hard edges'. (The names have since been added to the image by the therapist.) Jay was able to agree that the mark below the 'Thomas' triangle is reminiscent of a beating heart on monitor and, much later in therapy (review) saw that 'Simon' was a 'flat liner' and lifeless. At this stage, he recognised that the dissociated 'Thomas' element was in fact full of life as Jay the 'live wire' once was, whereas the square was boring, 'a square'.

A new voice, 'Alan', manifested some months into the work. Jay was not sure whether he was 'bad' or 'good' and indeed Jay's tendency to view others in absolute black and white terms was softening. The new voice was envisioned as a Norman arch, which is an effective visual combination of all elements of self: the triangle, square and circle. This implies a movement towards integration of his dissociated parts, though, subjectively for Jay, they remained 'other'. He was now working actively with the voices and made many figurative depictions of 'Thomas'. In Plate 9, 'Thomas' is abstracted and held within a margin. In Plate 10, he is more loosely drawn, without margin, and stands triumphant in the surrounding tempest.

Plate 11, made after some 22 months of art therapy, shows further progress towards the integration of dissociated material. The Jay element is more strongly drawn than the surrounding voices. All figures share the same geometric figuration and the voices are much less 'other'. The image resembles a Venn diagram. There is a clear overlap between Jay and the material that was previously wholly dissociated. In particular the 'bad' Thomas figure is marked with an arrow leading directly into the Jay figure. This suggests a direction the therapy subsequently followed: more conscious acceptance of responsibility for the murders and profound remorse. Of particular note is the casual spontaneous and exploratory sketch-like quality. This could not have occurred without the sense of containment provided by the therapeutic space.

Vignette 2: 'Grandma's pancake on Dad's head'

Plate 12 was made by a woman in her 50s who had suffered emotional deprivation and trauma as a child. At age four she was taken away from her alcoholic mother, to live with her non-English speaking paternal grandmother. The grandmother taught her to cook and otherwise service the needs of her father. Affect, when she described physical and sexual abuse, was flat. The kinaesthetic properties of clay helped her get in touch with repressed feelings. When she made the head of her father in clay, powerful emotions about the beatings and humiliations he had subjected her to, enlivened her. In turn, she beat and humiliated the clay head. It has thick lips, big mouth (he shouted), big nose (she had no privacy) and eyes pulled out (aged 14, she was made to walk topless in front of relatives to 'cure' her embarrassment at having breasts).

Suddenly she remembered that she had made a clay model for her father when she was a child, and that her gift, a work she treasured, had been used as a doorstop by her paternal grandmother. This brought up many more memories of humiliations and rejections. She rotated and stretched a small ball of clay in her hands. The clay was drawn out thinner and thinner as she recalled her suffering in a much more present way. At the end of the session, when she actually looked at the clay she was holding, she exclaimed: 'Grandma's pancake on Dad's head!' and banged it on the damaged clay head. This was a cathartic experience and for the first time in the therapy she laughed and felt empowered.

CONCLUSIONS

Art therapy is a flexible and wide-ranging intervention with a growing body of theory, its own literature, and a developing evidence base. It is now used widely in mental health services, for example it is recommended in the NICE guidelines on treatment for schizophrenia.

Although it is used for a range of difficulties it is most obviously useful for those who cannot express themselves easily in words, and for people who are excessively verbal. In both situations the discovery of a visual form of communication can be particularly helpful. Aspects of art therapy, such as image making and reflection on images, can be introduced to students as a form of experiential learning. It has been possible to give only a flavour of the theory and clinical practice of art therapy in this chapter, therefore further reading has been included.

Recommended reading

Adamson E. *Art as Healing: an illustrated account of the early pioneer stage of art therapy in a psychiatric hospital*. London: Coventure; 1984.

Campbell J (editor). *Art Therapy, Race and Culture*. London: Jessica Kingsley; 1988.

Case C, Dalley T (editors). *The Handbook of Art Therapy: an introduction to art therapy in theory and practice*. London: Routledge; 1992.

Connell C. *Something Understood: art therapy in cancer care*. London: Wrexham Publications; 1998.

Dalley T (editor). *Art As Therapy: general survey of art therapy in different contexts*. London: Tavistock; 1984.

Edwards D. *Art Therapy*. London: Sage Publications; 2004.

Hagood M. *The Use of Art in Counselling Child and Adult Survivors of Sexual Abuse*. London: Jessica Kingsley; 2000.

Hogan S. *Healing Arts: the history of art therapy*. London: Jessica Kingsley; 2001.

Levens M. *Eating Disorders and Magical Control of the Body: treatment through art therapy*. London: Routledge; 1995.

Liebman M. *Art Therapy with Offenders*. London: Jessica Kingsley; 1995.

Pratt M, Wood M (editors). *Art as Therapy in Palliative Care: the creative response*. London: Routledge; 1988.

Rees M. *Drawing on Difference: art therapy with people who have learning difficulties*. London: Routledge; 1988.

Sandle D. *Development and Diversity: new applications in art therapy*. London: Free Association Books; 1998.

Simon R. *The Symbolism of Style*. London: Routledge; 1992.

Skaife S, Huet V (editors). *Art Psychotherapy Groups: between pictures and words*. London: Routledge; 1998.

Waller D, Gilroy A (editors). *Art Therapy: a handbook*. Philadelphia, PA: Open University; 1992.

Waller D. *Becoming a Profession: history of art therapy in Britain 1940–1982*. London: Tavistock/Routledge; 1991.

REFERENCES

1 British Association of Art Therapists. Homepage. Available at: www.baat.org/art_therapy.html (accessed 8 June 2010).

2 Health Professions Council. Homepage. Available at: www.hpc-uk.org (accessed 15 May 2010).

3 Rank O. *Art and Artist: creative urge and personality development*. Reprint. New York, NY: Norton; 1989.

4 May R. *The Courage to Create*. 1st ed. New York, NY: Norton; 1975.

5 Stewart C. *The Symbolic Impetus: how creative fantasy motivates development*. 1st ed. London: Free Association Books; 2001.

6 Wollheim R. *Art and Its Objects*. 2nd ed. Cambridge: Cambridge University Press; 1980.

7 MacGregor J. *The Discovery of the Art of the Insane*. 1st ed. Princeton, NJ: Princeton University Press; 1989.

8 Harrison C, Wood P (editors). *Art in Theory 1900–1990: an anthology of changing ideas*. Reprint (paperback). Oxford: Blackwell; 2001.

9 Cardinal R. *Outsider Art*. 1st ed. London: Studio Vista; 1972.

10 Rodman S. *Conversations with Artists*. 1st ed. New York: Devin-Adair; 1957.

11 Elkins J. *The Domain of Images*. 1st ed. (paperback). New York: Cornell Paperbacks; 2001.

12 d'Errico F, Henshilwood C, *et al*. The search for the origin of symbolism, music and language: a multidisciplinary endeavour. *J World Prehist*. 2003; **17**(1): 1–70.

13 Lewis-Willams D. *The Mind in the Cave*. 1st ed. London: Thames & Hudson; 2002.

14 Gimbutas M. *The Goddesses and Gods of Old Europe 6500–3500BC: myths and cult images*. Reprint (paperback). London: Thames & Hudson; 1989.

15 Black R. *Old and New Australian Aboriginal Art*. 1st ed. Sydney: Angus & Robertson; 1964. Halifax J. *Shaman: the wounded healer*. Reprint (paperback). London: Thames & Hudson; 1997.

16 Wyman L. *Sandpaintings of the Navaho Shootingway and the Walcott Collection*. 1st ed. Washington, DC: Smithsonian Institution Press; 1970.

17 Schaverien J. *The Revealing Image: analytical art psychotherapy in theory and practice*. 1st ed. (paperback). London: Jessica Kingsley; 1991.

18 Calvino I. *Six Memos for the Next Millenium*. Paperback ed. London: Vintage; 1996.

19 Barthes R. *Mythologies*. Paperback ed. London: Vintage; 2000.

20 Langer S. *Philosophy in a New Key: a study in the symbolism of reason, rite and art*. 3rd ed. (paperback). Cambridge, MA: Harvard University Press, 1979.

21 Stevens A. *Ariadne's Clue: a guide to the symbols of humankind*. 1st ed. Harmondsworth: Allen Lane; 1998.

22 Bachelard G. *On Poetic Imagination and Reverie* (trans C Gaudin). 3rd ed. (paperback). Dallas, TX: Spring Publications; 1989.

23 Milner M. *On Not Being Able to Paint*. 1st ed. (paperback). Oxford: Heinemann Educational; 1971.

24 Rawson P. *The Art of Drawing: an instructional guide*. 1st ed. London: Macdonald; 1983.

25 Arnheim R. *Art and Visual Perception: a psychology of the creative eye*. 50th anniversary paperback ed. Berkeley, CA: University of California Press; 1974.

26 Maclagan D. *Psychological Aesthetics: painting, feeling and making sense.* 1st ed. London: Jessica Kingsley; 2001.

27 Thomson M. *On Art and Therapy: an exploration.* Paperback edition. London: Free Association Books; 1997.

28 Tuby M. A Jungian definition of symbols. *Inscape.* 1976; 13.

29 Case C, Dalley T. *The Handbook of Art Therapy.* London: Brunner-Routledge; 2002. p. 220.

30 Wood C. Facing fear with people who have a history of psychosis. *Inscape.* 1997: 41–8.

31 Winnicott DW. *Playing and Reality.* Harmondsworth: Pelican Books; 1974.

32 Morter S. Where words fail: a meeting place. In: Killick K, Schaverian J. *Art, Psychotherapy and Psychosis.* London: Brunner-Routledge; 2002. p. 220.

33 Bick E. The function of the skin in early object relations. In: Briggs A. *Surviving Space: papers on infant observation.* London: Karnac; 2003. pp. 55–71.

34 Luzzatto P, Gabriel B. Art Psychotherapy. In: Holland JC. *Psycho-oncology.* New York: Oxford University Press; 1998. pp. 743–56.

35 Gross R. *Psychology: the science of mind and behaviour.* New York: Oxford University Press; 1997.

36 Hinz L. *The Expressive Therapies Continuum.* 1st ed. (paperback). Abingdon: Routledge; 2009. p. 146.

37 Dubowski JK. Alternative models for describing the development of children's graphic work: some implications for art therapy. In: Dalley T. *Art as Therapy.* London: Brunner-Routledge; 1999. pp. 45–61.

38 Ehrenzweig A. *The Hidden Order of Art.* Paperback edition. London: Phoenix Press; 2000.

39 Cage J. *Colour and Meaning: art, science and symbolism.* 1st ed. London: Thames & Hudson; 1999.

CHAPTER 9

The aesthetics of mania: an introduction for health professionals

Rob van Beek

INTRODUCTION

The aim of this chapter is to facilitate discussion of mania and manic psychosis as aesthetic experiences, that is, as experiences that may be intrinsically rewarding and meaningful for the person who is experiencing them. In the humanities, various forms of criticism are used to discuss artworks and aesthetic phenomena. In this chapter, readers from a variety of mental health backgrounds are invited to consider some of the experiences of mania and manic psychosis from a viewpoint that is informed by the arts and philosophy. This chapter aims to encourage humanities-based discussions of mental health phenomena amongst groups of health professionals.

Mood swings are part of life. Everyone experiences highs and lows, mostly in response to life events. Many people reading this chapter will have experienced persistent low mood and will have first-hand experience of how mood influences ideas and feelings about past, present and future life. Other readers (like this author) may also have experienced persistent high moods, for which they may have been hospitalised and for which they may take long-term medication. Additionally, in a book for mental health professionals, almost all readers will have experience of working with people who have had, or who are in, extreme moods.

There has been a long and ongoing debate over the nature and status of 'mental health' and 'mental illness'. Even the appropriate way to talk about these issues is contested and controversial. This chapter is not concerned with these battles. Whatever the intellectual status of extreme psychological states, their capacity to cause suffering to the person experiencing them and to those close to them is undeniable. This distress is of course compounded by prejudice, fear and misunderstanding. In a broad sense, the aim here is to show that extreme and extraordinary experiences can be discussed as part of, and alongside, other features of our culture.

A FORMAT FOR GROUP DISCUSSIONS

I have tried to create a format that will enable mental health professionals to consider some experiences of mania from an aesthetic point of view.

Below are materials for four discussion groups A, B, C and D. These can be used in a variety of educational contexts to stimulate discussion. Each discussion group takes a topic that is first introduced as a medical symptom of mania and then as a personal experience and an aesthetic experience. These topics are Elevated Mood, Racing Thoughts, Confusion and Delusions. The recollected personal and aesthetic experiences are based on the author's own history of extreme mood swings. They are included because they *appear* to have certain aesthetic features or characteristics. The purpose of the discussions is to consider and engage with these experiences and to explore whether they really do have aesthetic features or characteristics. Although these examples are drawn from personal experience they are broadly consistent with both clinical observations and other personal accounts of mania. Elevated Mood is selected because it is widely taken as the 'driving force' behind manic experiences. Racing Thoughts can be one of the more minor phenomena of mood swings, while both Confusion and Delusions are clearly major and dramatic conditions. However, any of the standard clinical symptoms could have been taken as a starting point for discussion, i.e. grandiosity, increased activity, de-inhibition, impulsiveness, impaired judgement, euphoria, pressured speech or hallucinations.

Following the introduction of each topic one or two parallels between these experiences and some phenomena or features from the arts or aesthetic life are added. These comments are included to help participants relate the personal experiences of mania to broader artistic and aesthetic issues.

Finally, to facilitate a new and unfamiliar kind of discussion, some remarks from imaginary health professionals have been included. Participants in the discussions may want to agree, disagree or take issue with any of these contributions.

(At this juncture, it would probably be helpful to look ahead to the discussion group sections in order to understand the form they take and then return to the next section on critical approaches.)

CRITICAL APPROACHES

Criticism

It is sometimes tempting for people from scientifically informed disciplines to consider activities that do not claim to be scientific as somewhat arbitrary or lacking in rigour or method. In the humanities, however, research and criticism are not a matter of simply stating a personal judgement or preference. Criticism involves both knowledge of a given subject matter and the ability to use language to draw attention to key features and qualities of works, events and performances. Good criticism is salient, perceptive and original. Criticism is not an activity that somehow *fails* to become scientific or rigorous, but a different *kind* of activity. It is an activity in which people use their intelligence and sensitivity to explore their experience of the natural and cultural world.

Health professionals who take part in these group discussions are being asked to set aside their professional hats and discuss these phenomena firstly from a broad human and cultural point of view, as fellow human beings, but also as critics might discuss a film, a book or a city. This involves comparing the phenomena with other perhaps more familiar or commonly shared experiences. The key questions participants should be asking themselves are: If I were having this experience what would it be like? What other experiences would this resemble? And ultimately, are these kind of experiences aesthetic?

Philosophy

It will become apparent that these critical discussions very quickly become 'philosophical'. Philosophy is not so different from criticism. It provides an opportunity to think about topics and possibilities that may otherwise be overlooked or brushed aside in everyday practical life. The popular image of 'being philosophical' is of making sweeping generalisations or being resigned to circumstance. Philosophy is usually more practical, effective and analytical than this image suggests. For example, in the discussions that follow many 'theoretical' concepts such as 'subjective' or 'objective', 'real' or 'unreal', 'mental' or 'physical', will emerge. However, when in philosophical mode these concepts cannot simply be accepted or taken for granted. It is important to ask, 'real for whom?' and 'objective in what sense?' This is because there are different kinds of accounts or theories about what is 'mental' and what is 'physical' and also about what is 'objective' or 'subjective', 'real' or 'apparent'.

It is in the nature of philosophy to be questioning but it can also be very creative. Philosophy takes notice of the results produced by different scientific disciplines (for example, the philosophy of mind has a close interest in neuroscience). However, philosophy is free to produce arguments and points of view that can go well beyond what any scientifically produced evidence might suggest. Philosophy can consider what might be *logically* possible as well as what seems likely or probable.

Aesthetics

In universities the subject of philosophy is studied in various branches. The branch that addresses the nature of art, beauty and aesthetic experience is called 'philosophical aesthetics'. The range of topics studied in philosophical aesthetics is now quite wide and includes issues such as the nature of pictorial representation, literary narrative and natural beauty. Nevertheless, many of the core issues in aesthetics hinge on questions of value. Why do people value or appear to value some objects and experiences 'for their own sake'? Why is it that these preferences seem to be neither entirely conventional nor entirely personal? Aesthetics and aesthetic debate in turn influence criticism – for example it is natural to ask what the basis or criteria for critical judgements or evaluations are, and these questions lead to discussions that may have both practical and theoretical significance.

These remarks about criticism, philosophy and aesthetics are intended to give readers from a mental health background a few pointers about the culture of the humanities that they are entering. The following section takes the form of a critical discussion in which health professionals consider some phenomena taken as symptoms of mania as aesthetic experiences. The final section of this chapter considers some of the topics that come up in these discussion groups. These topics relate to some major themes in philosophy and aesthetics.

Discussion groups: A to D

In the following discussions definitions of symptoms broadly follow those given in diagnostic manuals. The accounts of symptoms as personal and aesthetic experiences are summaries of the author's own experiences. In 'viewpoint from the arts', the author has added some possible parallels between manic and specifically artistic phenomena to stimulate debate. The various 'contributors' to the ensuing discussions are imaginary and are presented as a way of stimulating group discussion.

Discussion Group A: Elevated Mood

As a symptom

When mood is elevated for more than a week it can be a symptom of a manic episode.

As a personal and aesthetic experience

'As someone who experiences mood swings I frequently have spells of elevated mood – perhaps once every couple of months. These usually settle down without much incident but very occasionally they spiral out of control. It always seems to be fine weather when I go high like this. I will feel happy and positive and I will look on the bright side of things. Everything seems to show its bright side back to me. Within a day, or even a few hours though, this high mood can turn into something else – a strangely rearranged way of thinking and experiencing the world. Anything, even rubbish or things I might normally find offensive, can strike me as extraordinarily beautiful or significant. If my mood continues to rise, objects will begin to become less solid and stable. I will tend to experience the world more as sensory qualities such as sounds, patterns, colours rather than as recognisable and separate objects. Ultimately, I can become lost in looking at these beautiful appearances. I remember looking at reflected patches of light and colour for what seemed to be hours. I felt that I was experiencing everything, including myself, not as separate objects but as flows of energy. Even now I look back at these moments as among the most beautiful, extraordinary and happiest of my life'.

A viewpoint from the arts

In the arts, the mood of individual works of art is set by an overall or pervasive tone or quality. For example, a painting may be dark or light in tone; a dance may be fast or slow. Persistent features suggest certain interpretations – very dark paintings are unlikely to be cheerful, fast dances are unlikely to be sad. All the arts seem to manipulate their overall tone or mood to suggest atmosphere and feeling. Once a certain mood or atmosphere has been created it becomes more likely that good or bad, happy or sad things should happen. Events can run with the general mood or atmosphere or run against them.

Mental health professionals discussion

i 'I know that if I am in a good mood it makes everything more cheerful. Equally if you go to somewhere depressing it *is* depressing. Whether you are manic or not, I think there is a link between mood and environment and between our environment and how we feel and think'.

ii 'An environment does not become more or less beautiful because of the mood you happen to be in. If he is suffering from a mood disorder it is likely that his responses will be out of step with reality and out of step with other peoples' responses'.

iii 'Who is to say what the "right" way to respond is? Tastes and values change rapidly. For example, if the Hippies had achieved world domination perhaps seeing everything as beautiful would be the "normal" or official way of looking at things'.

iv 'He is in a "Catch 22" situation. If people believe he is having manic experiences they are not going to believe him, whatever he says. If he is no longer manic and he says that those past experiences were beautiful, then people will say, "Well, that is how they appeared to you but you were not yourself then"'.

v 'I do not think that manic experience is isolated from ordinary experience in this respect. He points to the colour, pattern and other effects that his world is dissolving into. That is not incomprehensible. Nature is full of beautiful fleeting effects of light, colour and pattern. This is normal. This is just aesthetic experience'.

Discussion Group B: Racing Thoughts

As a symptom

'Racing thoughts' are often linked to 'pressured speech' as a symptom of hypomania or mania. One idea suggests another in a way that is barely logical or sequential. Racing thoughts are also associated with 'distractibility', which is another standard clinical symptom.

As a personal and aesthetic experience

'Perhaps once a month I experience some "speediness". Typically these periods settle down if I am careful about my sleep. However, I can find it hard to "switch-off" as new ideas and plans keep surfacing. This is a pleasant state to be in. When I am a bit speedy I tend to feel I am very intelligent and very witty. It may seem odd to think of *thinking* as an "aesthetic" phenomenon but to me there is a special joy in making new connections between ideas. When my thinking is like this I am struck by more coincidences than usual and begin to find puns and anagrams hidden in words, images and symbols. From bitter experience I know that the "connectedness" of speedy and racing thoughts comes at the price of accuracy and precision. As my thinking accelerates I may go into a full-blown manic episode. I will not be able to contain my racing thoughts or the new ideas they are generating. Experience will become unstable and fluid but within this maelstrom there are centres of peace and tranquility. It can feel wonderful to lose rigour, accuracy and let go of realism. In their place I have experienced unique moments, where everything has appeared relevant and connected to everything else'.

A viewpoint from the arts

Creativity is important in all spheres of human activity but is often given free reign in the arts. Racing thoughts and manic thinking appear to resemble some aspects of creative thought. For example, poetry makes creative use of language. Similarly, poetic language refers to the poet's thoughts and to the world but it also plays with language using rhyme and other forms of pattern and coincidence.

Mental health professionals discussion

i 'People manipulate the pace of their thinking all the time through drugs, exercise, computer games, gambling or just by socializing, for example. These things are pleasurable. They make life feel more intense. I do not see the difference between the pleasure in these kinds of activities and being speedy because you are a bit manic'.

ii 'He might think he is enjoying these racing thoughts but that is part of his illness. His thoughts are involuntary and increasingly out of his control. If he were not ill he would be very alarmed by these effects'.

iii 'There may be similarities between racing thoughts and creative thinking but creative thinking is also productive. Manic thinking usually only produces a humiliating comedown and a crash into depression'.

iv 'I think the issue of connectedness and unity is important. However, I would say this was a *spiritual* state of mind rather than an aesthetic one. There is more to life than lots of facts and details. It is important that people sometimes experience a sense of unity and oneness with the universe'.

v 'Maybe when we are babies there is only "unity" and the emotion of being part of everything around you. As we grow up and have to deal with practical life, we lose touch with "unity" although perhaps it is always there. Racing thoughts and the manic experiences that grow out of them may reconnect us with this earlier, more elementary, way of relating to the world'.

vi 'Theories are fine but at the end of the day you are dealing with someone who is psychotic. If these are "personal and aesthetic experiences" why do they disappear at the first sight of Haloperidol? These effects are pathological.'

Discussion Group C: Confusion (Time)

As a symptom

Confusion is a general term that refers to impaired cognitive performance. Perception, memory, reasoning and the ability to understand meaning can all be affected by elevated mood. This group discussion focuses on the confused experience of time that can be a symptom of mania.

As a personal and aesthetic experience

'I find it quite easy to lose track of time and become over-immersed in activities. If I am becoming a little high or speedy I have to check the time on my watch to make sure I am not overrunning or overfilling time. If my mood becomes distinctly high then my sense of duration and awareness of clock time becomes increasingly vague. Beyond this, I begin to experience zones of "presentness". These are rather like reflective or meditative states. I get a strong and tangible sense that time is artificial or constructed and timelessness is natural and enduring. As I become psychotic, temporal episodes can become really confused, out of sequence, compressed or extended. This can produce bizarre effects. For example, I have thought people who have left the room for a few minutes and come back, have been away for several hours! I have sat and watched a clock and been unable to see it move. Indeed, I have thought I could stop clocks and watches just by looking at them!

These quite extreme effects can create a barrier between myself and other people around me. This is because people are busy doing things *in time*. For me, inside the barrier, there is only "presentness" and this experience can be profoundly peaceful. Sometimes when I am in this state, I feel very close to people I have known but who are now dead. I can almost hear their voices and sometimes find myself talking and sharing jokes with them. I feel closer to the dead than the quick (living). It *feels* as if the state that I am in is a more serious and profound one than that inhabited by the people around me. Because of this feeling disagreements and conflicts can arise. Just because we share the same surroundings does not mean that we are in the same world'.

A viewpoint from the arts

Many art forms take liberties with time – films and novels can compress years and extend moments and they can skip back and forwards in time. In the same way, a piece of music can race or dawdle and make us experience the passing of time differently. Works of art and entertainment do not simply stop but have some form of culmination. At the end of a novel, film or piece of music, the overall meaning or effect of the piece usually becomes apparent.

Mental health professionals discussion

i 'When I finish a special book I feel both happy and sad. The end of a book is a culmination but it is also the end of a relationship that has taken me outside of everyday life. You could see mania as taking you outside of everyday life in a more drastic way – a way you cannot control or escape from. But maybe it can still have personal meaning and aesthetic characteristics for the person who has created and lived through it'.

ii 'Many people these days experience time as a source of stress. In comparison, being confused about time sounds like an escape, even a therapy. Perhaps, we should all have our sense of time uncoupled periodically – perhaps we do when we watch television, or go to see a film?'

iii 'Time does not exist. It is merely a useful convention. The confusion is ours not the person who is experiencing mania'.

iv 'I imagine that looking at things "out of time" is like looking at precious arte-facts in a museum. If you are manic you might be able to look at everything as complete and perfect, you do not have to change anything about it. At a given moment you can just accept the world for the wonder it is'.

v 'It is possible that we live in a science-fiction world where people's personalities do live on as "information in the ether". It could turn out that there are states of consciousness for talking to the dead and cracking jokes with them. In the future, our view of the universe may change. Instead of being seen as people who tried to help others in these states of consciousness – health professionals could be seen as their tormentors'.

Discussion Group D: Delusions

As a symptom

Delusions are normally characterised as 'false beliefs' or changes of belief that are strongly out of character for the individual concerned. They can be symptomatic of several conditions including mania.

As a personal and aesthetic experience

i 'If I become very high I will almost certainly experience delusions. I have expe-rienced delusions about particular situations and delusions that took the form of a radical change in my general outlook. An example of the former was when I thought, for no good reason, that someone I knew had been kidnapped. An example of the latter, was when I suddenly became very religious or mystical in outlook'.

ii 'In my experience delusions have a number of strongly contrasted qualities. My delusions were quite complicated but they seemed to come from nowhere, spontaneously. They immediately took the place of my previous beliefs and at the same time I was immediately and implacably attached to them. Like revela-tions they became the new bedrock of my world. Above all, delusions seem to have the power to *explain*: radical, general delusions seem to explain *everything*. Consequently, they impart a strong sense of *unity* or coherence. They are unifying stories or theories that seem to explain and harmonise everything'.

A viewpoint from the arts

People continually generate explanations and narratives about the situations they are in. These need not be realistic or true but they have at least to be satisfactory for the individual concerned. People are continually reinterpreting the situations they find themselves in and find it impossible to stop doing so. Even when we sit down in front of the television or go to the cinema we relax by interpreting and making sense of the information that is being presented to us. Less narrative art forms, such as painting, sculpture or music, also have a narrative dimension. For example, paintings often have religious messages or illustrate someone's everyday life.

Mental health professionals discussion

i 'I think the point about attachment to ideas and beliefs is important. Many people have fixed beliefs and cling to them despite any amount of evidence to the contrary. Why expect delusional people to be any different?'

ii 'We all make up stories about how we think things are. If you are manic, eventually you will make up manic stories about how the world is. There is no difference in principle here; it is just that manic stories tend to be disruptive for other people because they are so egocentric'.

iii 'Situations that you cannot make sense of are confusing, frustrating and frightening. If we can suddenly understand those situations they become clear. We feel a release from tension and that feels rewarding – that is why we enjoy stories, explanations and theories. If you are delusional you are in a very confusing world – you have to come up with bigger and better delusions to try to make sense of it. It is not surprising that people become emotionally attached to their delusions'.

iv 'People who are delusional are completely egocentric and cannot distinguish fact from fantasy. They cannot be persuaded that their version is mistaken'.

v 'Even if someone is living in a fantasy world and their behaviour is a problem for the people around them it does not mean that their experience cannot be unique and satisfying in some ways. If these experiences did not exist then humanity would be the poorer for it'.

Themes emerging from the discussion groups

In philosophy, relatively informal discussions and debates such as these rapidly grow more technical and specialist in character. Key points that emerge are linked to the major themes and theories in philosophy. For example, the issue of reality or realism surfaced at several points in the preceding discussions. Common sense tends to tell us that we experience the world through our senses in a more or less simple, direct and immediate way. In contrast, research and argument suggests that the way we experience the world depends on a complex set of biological, psychological and social processes.

A second traditional theme in philosophy that began to emerge in the discussion groups concerned personal identity. The traditional philosophical question asks: What are the essential characteristics that make a person who they are? If we change in various physical, intellectual and psychological ways over time how can we be the same person? In other words, what are the essential traits that define us as individual people? To take a pertinent example: If I am experiencing a manic episode how much am I really myself? What does 'myself' mean in this context? Also, if I am not fully 'myself', who or what am I? Traditional philosophical interest in questions of personal identity has informed many legal discussions of mental capacity. Systems of justice often accept that a person who commits a crime when they are deemed psychologically impaired cannot be held fully responsible for their actions.

A third traditional philosophical question, which has been a theme throughout this chapter is: What is aesthetic experience? Is there really any such thing? If there is, why does it figure in human experience and what distinguishes it from other kinds of experience? These are all major and difficult questions that have puzzled philosophers and others for generations.

These themes of realism, personal identity and aesthetic experience converge quite dramatically when we ask ourselves whether experiences of mania have an aesthetic character or dimension. 'When I am manic do I really experience the world aesthetically or am I losing touch with reality and with myself?' This formulation links the problem of aesthetic experience to that of realism and to that of personal identity. It implies that aesthetic experiences have to be real and not mistaken in some way. Is it possible for someone to be confused about the aesthetic characteristics they are experiencing? Can we lose our normal or true capacity for experiencing something as beautiful, pleasing or interesting? These questions appear to link aesthetic experience to that of personal identity. If my identity is undergoing some kind of change, shift or crisis, will my capacity for aesthetic experience be a part of that or will it be distinct from that? If I believe I have strong aesthetic experiences when I am manic, are these to be taken as aberrant experiences explained wholly in terms of my pathology?

Within the scope of this chapter I can only raise such questions. However, on the basis of my own experience and reflections I would make the following tentative observations.

My own experience of manic states encourages me to say that these experiences had a strongly aesthetic character. These experiences felt as real and tangible as any other experience. However, in retrospect I can confidently say that I was mistaken about many things. Having undergone cycles of mood swings many times I have noticed that the kinds of things that one is mistaken about are broadly factual issues and states of affairs. They are not 'mistakes' about what one finds attractive or unattractive, pleasing or displeasing. In retrospect, many of the experiences of mania that I thought beautiful or moving whilst manic I still regard as beautiful and moving when non-manic. I am inclined to think of my state of mind as confused but *not* my aesthetic perception. Indeed, I see my confused state of mind as having provided new thoughts and experiences for aesthetic perception.

These tentative observations invert our customary way of thinking about the status of facts and values. Normally, we think of factual features and experiences as stable, solid and continuous. These 'hard' features are considered to exist in a way that is largely independent of our minds. Other kinds of features and experiences, such as aesthetic properties (e.g. softness, grace, delicacy) are usually considered to be subjective or evaluative in character and as being more dependent on the mind of the beholder. From the examples of aesthetic experience in mania that I have offered for discussion, it is not hard to see how the traditional schema of facts and values are transformed.

In mania, it is the factual, objective features of the world that become increasingly unstable, ethereal, discontinuous and mind-dependent. Many facts and pieces of information go missing or are systematically reinterpreted. In mania many causes and effects no longer add up or correspond in a meaningful way. Delusions and confusion about time are examples of this. Progressively, a world that is usually experienced as solid and stable becomes increasingly unstable and in flux. Correspondingly, those features that are usually associated with subjectivity or the aesthetic curiosity become more prominent and all pervasive. Instead of feeling that life is lived in a stable factual world that has an aesthetic veneer or surface, life is lived in a transfigured world that is subjective and aesthetic to its core. In mania, far from descending into a world of complete chaos, one descends into another kind of world whose rules and rationale are both egocentric and strongly influenced by personal desire and a need for reassurance.

CLOSING REMARKS

In this chapter, I have tried to explore whether manic symptoms can also be considered as aesthetic experiences. More precisely, I have tried to explore whether they can be discussed both in psychiatric and cultural or philosophical terms. I hope this chapter and the discussions that arise from it prove interesting and worthwhile.

As a final thought, I would like to close by reconsidering what I have called the aesthetics of mania and personal identity. Every major mood swing is a psychological and social challenge to the identity of the individual involved. After every major crisis people have to recover and rebuild their worlds and their lives. The topics discussed encourage the view that there are aspects of our personalities that ensure that there is always something to rebuild on and to rebuild with. In other words, we can sometimes lose our capacity to deal with life but we never entirely lose those key capacities that make us the people we are.

CHAPTER 10

Learning about community arts

Theo Stickley and Kate Duncan

INTRODUCTION

In this chapter, we discuss the concept of 'community arts' and its relevance to mental health and education. Community arts in mental health is distinguished by the premise that people who engage with community-based arts programmes are participants in the creative process. Community arts is also known, therefore, as 'participatory arts'. More recently, this type of approach has been widely associated with the 'arts and health' agenda. This agenda is led by the Arts Council England and the Department of Health (DoH) and has gained great momentum in recent years.[1,2] Subsequently, we pay special attention to the mental health benefits of the arts and health within this agenda.

Community arts differ significantly from arts therapy, as there is no interpretive component. Community arts philosophy is centred on the notion that everybody is creative, anyone can be an artist and that participating in creative activities with other people is intrinsically good for us. Naturally, an evidence base has developed for this work, although it will invariably be disappointing to the more reductionist enquirer. The benefits of participation in the arts are often associated with things that are not so easily measured, such as self-esteem, confidence and friendship.

In this chapter we intend to introduce the reader to community arts and explain its significance in learning about mental health. The chapter includes:

➤ an insight into the historical development of community arts
➤ an introduction to the politics of community arts in the UK
➤ examples of what community arts looks like in practice
➤ some background information regarding arts and health research
➤ a rationale for participation as a philosophy for education
➤ some proposed learning outcomes.

A BRIEF HISTORY OF THE ARTS AND MENTAL HEALTH

Arts in mental healthcare had its origins in the moral treatment movement of the early nineteenth century.[3] Subsequently, art therapy grew in popularity in the early half of last century. It would not be until the 1970s, however, that the arts in healthcare would become recognised as a legitimate intervention. Whilst the following quotation may, at first reading, have a strong egocentric component, the author's assertion is hard to refute:

> The 'Arts in Health Care' movement in this country can be said to have started in 1973 when I was given permission to become artist in residence at St Mary's Hospital, Manchester.[4]

Prior to this date, the arts had been awarded little attention in the National Health Service (NHS) in the UK other than in the context of architectural design and paintings on the walls; the notion of therapeutic space came later.[5] The earliest government attention given to the arts in healthcare can be found in a DoH report called *Art in the NHS*.[6] Two years later, this was followed by the Attenborough Report, specifically addressing the needs of people with disabilities.[7] In 1988, the DoH published *Arts and Healthcare*, which laid the foundations for the development of the arts in health.[8] The subsequent decade saw in the era of New Labour and with this a developing connection between the arts (and sport) and 'neighbourhood renewal'.

In the *Report of the Policy Action Team 10* (PAT 10), it was argued that participation in the arts and sport would help to improve a community's performance on the four identified key indicators of neighbourhood renewal: health, crime, employment and education.[9] However, the report observed that whilst there was much anecdotal evidence of the effectiveness of the arts and sports promoting community development, there was little research evidence. In its response to PAT 10, the Arts Council concurred that the arts could indeed contribute to the social inclusion agenda.[10] Another key event around this time was the Windsor Conferences (1998–99) organised by the Nuffield Trust. The focus of these events was to explore the potential of the arts in contributing to healthcare and therapy, health professional training, hospital design, and the promotion of healthy communities.[11]

The Health Development Agency (HDA) published the results of its national survey reviewing 'good practice in community-based arts projects and initiatives which impact upon health and well-being'.[12] The report acknowledges: 'Evidence for these benefits was predominantly anecdotal and no projects had designed rigorous instruments of measurement'.[12] Attempts at 'rigorous instruments of measurement' would come later with the implementation of the Department for Culture, Media and Sport (DCMS) programme in 2005.

In 2000, the first national focal point for arts and health was established, the National Network for the Arts and Health.[13] In 2003, a seminar was organised by the Institute for Public Policy Research (IPPR) and hosted by the DCMS. The agenda for this seminar included a discussion on the future of the arts and mental health in the UK. An overview of the national picture of the arts and mental health in the UK, especially in relation to social inclusion, was presented.[14]

The arts and mental health, in terms of its social inclusion agenda, was given a mandate for action on that day. Subsequently, the DCMS call for proposals to nationally research the arts and mental health was made. This work would build upon the Social Exclusion Unit Report on mental health and social exclusion.[15] Also, in 2004, the Arts Council (a UK government body) published its own research into the social benefits of engagement in the arts by examining participation in various funded projects.[16] This study reports a list of benefits of engagement with arts. However, as much of the research was conducted on behalf of the Arts Council, which also funded the majority of the projects, there were some questions regarding the validity of the research. Thus, the arts and mental health agenda had, for the first time, become nationally recognised at governmental level.

The government's White Paper *Choosing Health*[17] made no reference to the arts and health agenda, yet its progress continued with a report on the relationship between the arts and health.[18] These policy developments have grown in tandem with those specifically addressing people with mental health problems through the Office of the Deputy Prime Minister's Social Exclusion Unit.[15] In this report, the arts (and sport) have been identified as useful in promoting good health through social inclusion. Simultaneously, the Arts Council commissioned two reviews of the literature regarding the arts and health.[19,20] Staricoff included a section devoted specifically to mental health.[20] Furthermore, the Arts Council included a commitment to developing strategies on arts and health.[21] This was followed by two further policies endorsing the arts and health: *Arts, Health and Well-being* and the *Report of the Review of Arts & Health Working Group*.[1,2]

THE POLITICS OF COMMUNITY ARTS IN THE UK

When the Council for the Encouragement of Music and the Arts (later to become the Arts Council) was set up in 1940, it was required to choose whether it would support the creation of art by the population (community arts) or provide art displays and exhibitions for the people. It chose the latter. According to the Arts Council, art should be available to all the population through displays and exhibitions. This was further endorsed in 1956 by the then Secretary General of the Arts Council, WE Williams:

> The Arts Council believes then that the first claim upon its attention and assistance is that of maintaining in London and the larger cities effective power houses of opera, music and drama; for unless these quality institutions can be maintained, the arts are bound to decline into mediocrity.[22]

Art, therefore, was considered something that could be provided by the state for its people; thus the Arts Council openly declared its elitist origins. By the 1980s, resources were stretched to the extent that the Arts Council only funded professional artists. In spite of the existence of art therapy for decades, prior to the first document on the relationship between art and health, the link between the Arts and Health only became apparent in policy, following the election of New Labour in 1997. This should not be surprising, as there was no research agenda linking the arts with deprived areas experiencing high rates of illness. Matarasso heralded the arrival of New Labour optimistically:

> The election of a government committed to tackling problems like youth unemployment, fear of crime and social exclusion is the right moment to start talking about what the arts can do for society.[23]

Graef, a criminologist, asserts that artistic expression encompasses feelings that do not harm other people, but transforms the experience of both the giver and the receiver and enhances people's lives instead of damaging them.[24] Graef's thesis argues well for community arts in deprived inner city areas (for example, *see* Plate 13). As an alternative recent history has suggested:

> Perhaps if the fledgling Arts Council had decided, at that crucial, never-to-come-again moment at the end of the second world war, that community art was its remit, not showpiece art, the whole history of post-war Britain and all our preconceptions about what art is, would have been different.[22]

However, Matarasso encourages forward thinking as he claims that Britain deserves better than 'exhausted prejudices over post-war debates over state support for the arts' (p. 5).[23] There remains the potential for the arts to become another form of palliative therapy in the way that counselling has become mainstream in statutory healthcare provision, thus avoiding the responsibility for addressing underlying social needs. By 2000, the government had committed itself to an art and health agenda that specifically recognised the value of community arts in its review of good practice.[12] Whilst this is supported by policy frameworks, there remains a lack of financial commitment from government departments to fund the arts and health nationally.[1,25] At the time of writing there are numerous challenges to the arts and health agenda: a serious economic downturn, cuts in public spending, and significantly, Britain is focusing upon preparation for the 2012 Olympics. All this reveals that the arts and health agenda is very much subject to political pressure.

TWO EXAMPLES OF COMMUNITY ARTS PROJECTS

Case Study 1: Arts In-Reach

Mental health services in England are experiencing a period of unprecedented change. The focus of mental healthcare has shifted from asylums into the community with 90% of all mental healthcare provision in the UK being community-based. However, inpatient provision is still the focus of the greatest proportion of expenditure with regard to the adult mental health budget and employs the greatest number of staff.[26] Funding, therefore, is allocated predominantly to statutory service provision.

The Arts In-Reach programme of work focuses on delivering arts activities on six of the Treatment and Therapy (formally known as acute) wards in Nottinghamshire. The inpatient service provides care in times of crisis and offers a safe and therapeutic setting for service users. This scheme brings professional artists and arts assistants on to the wards for weekly workshops. The ethos of the programme is to provide an opportunity for participants to learn new arts-based skills. The programme also focuses on helping people to re-establish supportive social networks once they leave hospital. Lack of social support can lead to isolation and recurring ill health. The programme aims to address this by enabling service users to access community arts-based opportunities. Research is being conducted to assess the impact of the project on people's lives.

Case Study 2: Arts on Prescription

Arts on Prescription has developed jointly between NHS Trusts and a community arts organisation, City Arts (Nottingham) Ltd. The project was inspired by one of the original programmes, Stockport Arts on Prescription, which was established in 1995 and has since become a national example of best practice.[27] In 2004, the programme launched with artists delivering Poetry in the Waiting Room within four local health centres and weekly arts activities within the treatment and recovery wards at a local inpatient unit.

The scheme aims to offer support to people who are affected by mental health issues and offers creative ways of overcoming emotional difficulties and the daily stresses associated with ill health. This programme is positioned to complement mainstream interventions such as medication. Those attending include individuals experiencing stress, anxiety, grief and a wide range of mental health problems. Referrals are made to the programme by a range of health professionals. Weekly arts activities are delivered by professional artists, who have counselling skills and experience of art therapy. To offer consistency the same artists and arts assistants also work on the Arts In-Reach programme. The activities offered are as broad as possible, including creative writing, music, batik, photography, drawing and painting, textiles, mono printing and sculpture, (*see* Plate 14). Research is underway to assess the impact of this programme and will include service users as active stakeholders in the evaluation process.

BACKGROUND TO ARTS AND HEALTH RESEARCH

While the 'arts' are widely accepted as a form of therapy, their usefulness in promoting health to the general population remains largely unacknowledged in the healthcare arena and within its allied research base. The DoH claims that there are over 1000 studies supporting the health benefits of the arts, although the same document acknowledges that the majority of these are more to do with hospital environments than participation.[2] Specific research into the arts, creativity and its benefits for physical and mental health is in its infancy, being in a hypothesising/ generating stage.[28]

Whilst there has been much research regarding the efficacy of arts groups led by arts professionals,[29–33] there is little research into the benefits to people engaging with community arts, in spite of policy support.[1,25]

The benefits of community arts are reported in government commissioned research in response to the Social Exclusion Unit's reports on mental health and social exclusion: *Mental Health, Social Inclusion and Arts: developing the evidence base.*[34] The results suggested that there were significant improvements in empowerment, mental health and social inclusion related to involvement in community arts. The research indicates that arts projects can benefit people with a range of mental health needs, including those with significant mental health difficulties.

It has been suggested that social capital is increased following engagement with community arts, for example social well-being in terms of forming and sustaining relationships with other participants.[35]These results strengthen the 'bonding' personal capital argument for community arts.[36]

The social and well-being benefits of community arts have also been identified by Fisher and Specht with older people, and Reynolds and Prior with women coping with disability.[29,31] Whilst research on the arts and community engagement might be in its infancy, research examining the relationship between arts and health suggests many benefits to health related to engagement with the arts. For example, in her review of the Arts and Health literature, Staricoff identified beneficial outcomes, such as reduced drug consumption, shorter hospital stays and improved doctor-patient relationships.[20]

It is suggested that evaluation studies of community-based participation projects provide inconclusive evidence of effectiveness due to methodological difficulties.[37]

AN EDUCATIONAL PHILOSOPHY FOR PARTICIPATION

Naturally, community arts demands participation. There are also educational philosophies that emphasise the significance of participation. The need to participate in education is essential for more than mere intellectual development. Working with people with mental health problems requires emotional as well as intellectual understanding. It is widely understood that emotional learning takes place through experience and reflection.[38] This kind of learning has become known as 'experiential learning'.[39] Whilst much of psychiatric and mental health education might be devoted to developing the 'rational' mind, there is less emphasis given to the development of the 'emotional' mind. The notion of developing one's emotional intelligence has been popularised by Goleman, in his best selling book *Emotional Intelligence.*[40] Student participation in arts activities is one way of facilitating this type of intelligence. Fundamental to the concept of participation is the belief that the rational mind and the emotional mind need to be balanced; where this relationship is harmonious, intellectual ability increases and, we would argue, a deeper, more meaningful understanding of mental health problems will be developed. It might also be helpful to consider the notion that we have multiple intelligences.

Mental health education should incorporate approaches that appeal to the various forms of intelligence, including spatial capacity, musical, verbal and mathematical.[41] The arts may contribute to individual learning and growth by stimulating various types of intelligence. With its shift toward the academic, however, mental health education leans more towards the scientific paradigm and away from the emotional. A focus upon developing emotional intelligence through creative expression is one way of helping to develop a more balanced approach to mental healthcare.

At the heart of community arts delivery is the centrality of the participation of the recipient. This philosophy is consistent with the development of service user and carer involvement in healthcare and health education. Whilst this may not be as well developed in psychiatry, it is well established in nursing and social care.[42] We would argue that genuine involvement of people who use mental health services will inevitably promote emotional intelligence amongst learners. By listening to the voices of those who experience the distress of mental health problems and the associated stigma and discrimination, our hearts are moved by human experience. Additionally where curricula and specific modules are informed by service user experience and involvement, there will inevitably be a focus upon qualities and values that inform good practice.

For students of mental health, we would argue therefore that participation in the arts is essential in order to further understanding of the significance of community arts for people who are often marginalised by society. By engaging with the artistic expression of those who experience mental distress and subsequent exclusion, the student can develop an emotional understanding of the person's experiences.

COMMUNITY ARTS IN THE FUTURE

In recent times, community arts has become known as participatory arts and is strongly associated with the arts and health agenda. It might be that its future depends upon the significance of the impact these forms of arts have on the health of the nation. It is widely accepted that arts and health projects are largely funded through non-statutory sources; this in turn allows for a certain amount of flexibility and freedom with regard to the models of practice that often follow social rather than medical models. In spite of policy frameworks and public support from politicians, it has to be acknowledged that without direct funding from mainstream services, there still remains little public commitment from within the health sector. Subsequently, sustainability of projects will always be an issue. If current UK government policy to promote choice to individuals as a mechanism to promote change in services continues, funding may be provided directly from the consumer of health services. *New Horizons: towards a shared vision for mental health* aims to help shape mental healthcare services for the future and intends to build upon the National Service Framework in supporting the move towards more personalised services.[43,44] The outcome of this will identify the key priorities for ensuring that mental health commissioning delivers improved outcomes for service users, and offers participants the opportunity to help shape this model. This approach should improve opportunities for arts and health commissioning in the future.

Community arts have much to offer society in the future. This chapter has not attempted to summarise all the research on the health and social benefits of participatory arts; there is a growing literature on the subject and the reader is encouraged to access this and appreciate what impact the arts may have on people's lives. We have illustrated how through project delivery, community arts can connect with the needs of people that choose to participate. Taking part in community-based arts activities may bring joy and a sense of well-being, but the arts will never solve deep-rooted social problems. Whilst we strongly advocate for the arts and health agenda, it is no substitute for much-needed political solutions for the causes of people's problems.

For students of psychiatry and mental health, we would encourage engagement with the arts and humanities in order to appreciate the artistic elements of healing and we would urge students to engage with people who use mental health services and ask them what benefits the arts can give. It is this act of listening that can bring about true experiential learning. We would also urge students to take part. To find out for themselves what it is like to paint, draw, dance, write poetry and so on with other people. It is in the participation itself that transformation takes place; whether for healing or learning or both.

REFERENCES

1 Arts Council England. *Arts, Health and Well-being.* Arts Council England, London; 2007.
2 Department of Health. *Report of the Review of Arts and Health Working Group.* Crown, London; 2007.
3 Digby A. *Madness, Morality, and Medicine: a study of the York Retreat, 1796–1914.* New York, NY: Cambridge University Press; 1985.
4 Senior P. The arts in health movement. In: Kaye C, Blee T. *The Arts in Health Care: a palette of possibilities.* London: Jessica Kingsley; 1997. pp. 21–3.
5 Lynch J. Spaces between buildings in the healthcare estate. In: Kaye C, Blee T. *The Arts in Health Care: a palette of possibilities.* London: Jessica Kingsley; 1997. pp. 79–104.
6 Coles P. *Art in the National Health Service.* London: DHSS; 1983.
7 Carnegie Council. *Arts and Disabled People: the Attenborough Report.* London: Bedford Square Press; 1985.
8 Moss L. *Arts and Healthcare.* London: Department of Health; 1988.
9 Department for Culture Media and Sport. *Arts and Sport: Policy Action Team 10. A report to the Social Exclusion Unit.* London: Department for Culture, Media and Sport; 1999.
10 Arts Council England. Social exclusion: a response to Policy Action Team 10 from the Arts Council of England. Unpublished. London: Arts Council of England; 2000.
11 Clift S. Guest editorial: Arts and health. *Health Educ J.* 2005; **105**(5): 328–31.
12 Health Development Agency. *Art for Health.* London: Health Development Agency, HMSO; 2000.
13 Dose L. National network for the arts in health: lessons learned from six years of work. *The J R Soc Promo of Health.* 2006; **126**: 110.
14 White M, Angus J. *Arts and Adult Mental Health Literature Review.* CAHHM, University of Durham; 2003.

15 Social Exclusion Unit. *Mental Health and Social Exclusion.* London: Office of the Deputy Prime Minister, Social Exclusion Unit; 2004.

16 Jermyn H. *The Art of Inclusion.* London: Arts Council England; 2004.

17 Department of Health. *Choosing Health: making healthy choices easier.* London: HMSO; 2004.

18 Cowling J. *For Art's Sake? Society and the arts in the 21st century.* London: Institute for Public Policy Research; 2004.

19 Reeves M. *Measuring the Economic and Social Impact of the Arts: a review.* London: Arts Council England; 2001.

20 Staricoff RL. *Research Report 36. Arts in Health: a review of the medical literature.* London: Arts Council England; 2004.

21 Arts Council England. *Corporate Plan 2003–06.* London: Arts Council England; 2003. Available at: www.artscouncil.org.uk/publication_archive/corporate-plan-2003-2006-summary/ (accessed 15 May 2010).

22 Carey J. *What Good are the Arts?* London: Faber & Faber; 2005.

23 Matarasso F. *Use or Ornament? The social implication of participation in the arts.* Stroud: Comedia Publications; 1997. Available at: www.deveron-arts.com/wb/media/pdfs/OrnamentMatarasso.pdf (accessed 15 May 2010).

24 Graef R. The value of arts in prison. In: *Including the Arts: the route to basic and key skills in prisons.* London: The Home Office Standing Committee for Arts in Prisons; 2001. pp. 26–54

25 Department of Health and Arts Council England. *A Prospectus For Arts and Health.* London: Department of Health and Arts Council England; 2007.

26 Department of Health. *Mental Health Policy Implementation Guide Adult Acute Inpatient Care Provision.* London: Department of Health; 2002. p. 3.

27 Huxley PJ. *Arts on Prescription.* Stockport: Stockport NHS Trust; 1997.

28 Reynolds F. The effects of creativity on physical and psychological well-being: current and new directions for research. In: T Schmid (editor). *Promoting Health Through Creativity.* London: Whurr Publishers; 2005. pp. 112–31.

29 Fisher B, Specht D. Successful aging and creativity in later life. *J Aging Stud.* 1999; **13**: 457–72.

30 Reynolds F. Managing depression through needlecraft creative activities: a qualitative study. *Arts Psychother.* 2000; **27**: 107–14.

31 Reynolds F, Prior S. 'A lifestyle coat-hanger': a phenomenological study of the meanings of artwork for women coping with chronic illness and disability. *Disabil Rehabil.* 2003; **25**(14): 785–94.

32 Schmid T. *Promoting Health Through Creativity.* London: Whurr Publishers; 2005.

33 Greaves CJ, Farbus L. Effects of creative and social activity on the health and well-being of socially isolated older people: outcomes from a mutely-method observational study. *JRSH.* 2006; **126**(3): 134–42.

34 Anglia Ruskin University and the University of Central Lancashire. *Mental Health, Social Inclusion and Arts: developing the evidence base. Final report from Stage 1: the state of art in England.* Norwich: The APU/UCLAN Research Team, University of East Anglia; 2007.

35 Parr H. Mental health, the arts and belongings. *Trans Inst Br Geogr.* 2006; **31**(2):

150–66.

36   Putnam R. *Bowling Alone: the collapse and revival of American community.* New York, NY: Simon & Schuster; 2000.

37   Staricoff RL. Arts in health: the value of evaluation. *JRSH.* 2006; **126**(3): 116–20.

38   Schön D. *The Reflective Practitioner: how professionals think in action.* San Francisco: Jossey Bass; 1983.

39   Kolb DA. *Experiential Learning: experience as the source of learning and development.* Englewood Cliffs, NJ: Prentice Hall; 1984.

40   Goleman D. *Emotional Intelligence.* New York: Bantam; 1995.

41   Gardner H. *Frames of Mind.* New York: Basic Books Inc; 1983.

42   Rush B. Mental health service user involvement in England: lessons from history. *J Psychiatr Ment Health Nurs.* 2004; **11**: 313–18.

43   Department of Health. *New Horizons: towards a shared vision for mental health.* London: Department of Health; 2009.

44   Department of Health. *The National Service Framework for Mental Health.* London: Department of Health; 1999.

CHAPTER 11

The use of drama and theatre arts in mental health education

Victoria Tischler

The play's the thing
Wherein I'll catch the conscience of the king.

Hamlet[1]

INTRODUCTION

As a teacher of up to 260 medical students at a time I have found it important to provide a *performance* which elicits and maintains interest. I write this chapter from an educational perspective and as someone with an enthusiasm for drama and performance. I have taken acting classes but I do not profess to be an actor or professionally trained in theatre or drama. I have a musical background through singing, recording and performing some years ago through which I learnt voice projection skills, breathing control and dance. Acting classes have introduced me to roles such as William's Blanche Dubois in *A Streetcar Named Desire* and Mrs Cheveley in Wilde's *An Ideal Husband*. I have found that acting has enhanced my teaching, for example, in terms of vocal expression and breathing control, facilitating a more confident and assured delivery.

As health professionals and educators we adopt roles every day, that is, we conform to certain behaviours, dress a certain way and we use our own language (or jargon). Patients also adopt roles, for example the sick role which involves exemption from usual duties and a commitment to try to return to full health.[2] Acting can be used to introduce students to a variety of roles, to 'try them on' and to consider others' physicality, experiences and feelings.

Role play is routinely used in medical education but it is criticised for being 'unreal' and difficult for students with no acting background.[3] It is a limited medium, as students can participate in a superficial sense without ever really considering the impact of their professional role on the patient's experience or truly empathising with the patient. In contrast, drama involves action, engaging a person physically, emotionally and mentally,[4] as such it promotes experiential learning, impacting on learners at both an intellectual and emotional level.[5] In this way, it may be viewed as cathartic and also as an effective coping mechanism for mental health professionals dealing with human distress, often on a daily basis. Acting provides a medium for inhabiting the world of a patient or clinician and to deepen understanding of their experiences. Performance can help doctors develop their empathetic imagination, 'a cognitive skill set which helps to imagine the experiences and responses of another person' (p. 159).[6] Drama practice also provides useful transferable skills within and outside clinical practice, such as effective communication, vocal control and increased confidence. This chapter describes the design and delivery of drama sessions for medical students, illustrating with a teaching model that I and colleagues have developed.

MATERIALS FOR USE

The primary resources required are experienced actors and space. I have developed good working relationships with local actors who are also experienced teachers of health professionals. They understand the educational context, are confident in working with students who have no previous acting experience, and with issues related to clinical practice. Sessions pair actors with interested clinicians so that acting and clinical knowledge are combined. As discussed elsewhere in this volume, the participation of clinical staff in sessions is valued by students and provides positive role modelling.

Regular seminar rooms are not usually suitable for this type of teaching. Space is required so that participants can move around freely, make noise, and work in pairs or small groups. Teaching rooms can be adapted by moving chairs and tables to create space but it is better to use performing arts venues elsewhere on campus as they provide a conducive atmosphere with adequate space and soundproofing. It is also useful to have a video camera available for filming performances. A DVD recording can be reviewed by the group or individually and also acts as a form of evidence for portfolios and continuing professional development (CPD) activities.

SESSION PLANNING

Pre-meetings with acting and teaching staff allow for session objectives to be discussed, clarified and adapted as necessary. I have found that a series of linked workshops is effective for this teaching (*see* Table 11.1). This allows time for students to familiarise themselves with acting techniques, to have adequate rehearsal time, and to work towards a performance. The linked sessions are scheduled with several days between each allowing students to complete research and preparation required and to consolidate learning. Each session lasts 2–3 hours enabling sufficient time for performance, reflection and breaks.

TABLE 11.1 Acting session plan

Session 1	Session 2	Session 3
Games and warm ups	Games and warm ups	Games and warm ups
Improvisation scenarios	Feedback on character development	Rehearsal with directorial input
Character building including clinical guidance on accurate portrayal of symptomatology	Improvisation in character including interactions between characters	Performance filmed
Students chose characters/illness and given research tasks for next session	Plan for performance in next session	Feedback from performers

SETTING BOUNDARIES

It is essential to establish boundaries for the sessions to run smoothly and for students to feel able to participate fully. This includes ensuring confidentiality and appropriate follow-up in the event that a student becomes distressed. Given the nature of acting and the embodiment required, it can at times uncover issues of a sensitive and or personal nature which may require intervention. Given the commonplace nature of mental health problems, it is likely that students, their family or friends will have experienced mental distress at some time. Participants may be asked to draw upon personal experience, so they need to feel safe in order to explore this. Group exercises and 'warm ups' help build trust amongst participants.

TECHNIQUE AND SKILLS TRAINING

Students are introduced to a range of acting techniques and the philosophy behind each is explained in simple terms. Examples of well-known exponents are used; Augusto Boal and Konstantin Stanislavski are introduced here, and students are encouraged to undertake their own research if they wish to explore particular acting techniques in more depth.

Forum theatre was developed by Augusto Boal (1931–2009), a Brazilian-born theatre director. His aim was political: to use theatre as a means of social change. He challenged the dominance of the ruling elite in the theatre world and promoted the use of theatre as a mode by which the underprivileged could improve their lives.[7] This is achieved by the audience moving from passive spectator to active participant via direction or acting. For example, they can interrupt the play, and can 'direct' by suggesting what should happen next. They may also join the actors on stage and act themselves, thus exerting control over the course of the play. This format has been widely used in the health arena including with service users and mental health themes, so it can be easily adapted for teaching.

Konstantin Stanislavksi (1863–1938) is often referred to as the father of realism in theatre. He devised a system of external and internal actor training incorporating 'incarnation' and 'experiencing' respectively. These aspects, involving daily training (termed 'habits'), for example in vocal and breathing techniques, aim to ensure that acting performances are imbued with spiritual and emotional depth and that they do not become stale.[8] This approach emphasises the 'being' rather than 'playing', which is what differentiates acting from role play. Students may be introduced to this system via research and rehearsal; for example, they can be asked to research a character that they are playing. This includes identifying the overall objective of the play/act/scenario and how this relates to the character. A small section of text may be used to identify the character's objectives and actions (relating to that objective) and these are recorded in written form and discussed before rehearsing the scene. This type of textual analysis moves the actor beyond reading and towards the embodiment or 'being' that Stanislavski advocates.

I illustrate this technique using the example of the character of Blanche Dubois in *A Streetcar Named Desire*. The play depicts the tragic downfall of Blanche, a woman who has experienced a range of traumatic events involving financial and emotional losses, disgrace, betrayal and bereavement and, during the play, sexual assault at the hands of her brother-in-law. She seeks refuge with her sister Stella and brother-in-law, Stanley, but is eventually committed to an asylum by Stanley and a complicit Stella. How does this affect Blanche? She is proud in the face of adversity, increasingly vulnerable with age and losing touch with reality. This is revealed as she clings to the status of her gentrified past as a beautiful, youthful southern belle and a respectable teacher. She finds solace in the soft light of a paper lantern that conceals her true age, and the routine of her *toilette*, (involving washing, perfuming and dressing) in an attempt to maintain her role despite the derision of Stanley and a brief but doomed relationship with Stanley's friend, Mitch. I focus on a section in the final scene of the play. Blanche busies herself with her toilette, believing that an old beau (Shep Huntleigh) is calling for her. In fact, Stanley has arranged for her to be committed to an asylum. Blanche speaks:

> I can smell the sea air. The rest of my time I'm going to spend on the sea. And when I die, I'm going to die on the sea . . . I will die – with my hand in the hand of some nice-looking ship's doctor, a very young one with a small blond moustache and a big silver watch.[9]

Here the objective is to reveal Blanche's resignation and acceptance of her fate, yet also a sense of hope and fantasy that she will be rescued. This is revealed in Blanche's language, which is poetic, morbid, and also by her physical state, which appears weak, hesitant and on the verge of hysteria.

CLINICIAN INVOLVEMENT

Students may have limited clinical experience; so clinicians are involved in sessions to explain symptomatology and aetiology of mental disorders and to clarify factual details, such as representation of particular disorders, available treatments and clinical interventions. This ensures that characterisations and settings are realistic and that the sessions have clinical relevance. Students are encouraged to draw on their own personal or clinical experiences. Clearly this may arouse emotions, hence the importance of boundaries, as discussed previously. Anonymous case examples can be provided to describe how individuals may present using the mental state examination (MSE) checklist (*see* Box 11.1).[10] The students then build characters from these descriptions, guided by facilitators.

BOX 11.1 The mental state examination checklist

1. Appearance and behaviour
2. Speech
3. Mood plus risk assessment
4. Thought
5. Perception
6. Cognition
7. Insight

RUNNING THE SESSION

After introductions, the students are given a brief (*see* Box 11.2). Acting games and exercises are included at the start and throughout each session. Interested readers may wish to refer to Boal's text *Games for Actors and Non-actors*. The exercises reinforce the participative nature of the sessions. A selection of suggested exercises are included (*see* Table 11.2). The exercises are grouped under a particular focus for reference but perform multiple functions. They create energy and movement, promote interaction, foster cooperation and enhance voice projection. In addition the exercises relax students and relieve them of inhibitions. Educators join in with students to model participation, as noted earlier, and usually start/lead the exercises so that participants can see what to do in conjunction with hearing the instructions.

BOX 11.2 Brief for drama sessions

In session 3 we will be performing a 25-minute party scene. A group of individuals, each with a particular mental health diagnosis, will be attending the party. You will chose a character and research their illness/problem in detail. You will then act the part of the character in the party scene. The scene will be filmed and reviewed as a group.

Choose a particular psychiatric disorder that interests you. Research the condition in detail, noting aetiology, symptoms and behaviours, likely treatments and prognosis. Think about how you would depict that character through acting. Ask yourself the following questions: how might the person walk, talk, think and feel? How would they interact with others?

As a group we will write a script to guide the party scene. You will also be involved in direction of the piece. We will discuss the scene after filming and you will be given a copy of the film to keep.

Screenwriting exercises include building characterisation, using information including personal experience, knowledge and the MSE checklist, and devising a narrative, setting and dialogue for the characters. This approach can be adapted and a 'loose' script can work well, with actors improvising whilst in role for a more naturalistic approach. Students also discuss and delegate tasks including setting the scene, props, costume, and make up in preparation for the performance and filming session. Facilitators usually adopt the directorial and filming roles and lead feedback sessions post-rehearsal and performance. If the group is large, splitting them into smaller groups of three to six can be effective. It is therefore important to have at least two to three facilitators per session. Each session ends with an exercise (*see* Table 11.2 for suggestions) and students are given tasks to complete before the following session.

TABLE 11.2 Drama exercises

Focus	Suggested exercises
Warming up	*Last one standing*
	Participants stand in a circle. A chair is removed so there is one less chair than there are participants. Someone is selected to go to the centre of the circle and describe a characteristic about themselves which others may share, for example, 'anyone with pierced ears' or 'anyone who drank fruit juice today', 'anyone who went to the theatre last week'. Participants who 'match' or share that characteristic must stand and swap seats with one of the others who is also standing. The last person standing, that is, the one without a chair, continues by describing something about themselves and so on until all have had a turn in the centre of the circle.
	My animal
	Participants stand in a circle. Each person chooses an animal to imitate. One person (usually a facilitator) starts by imitating (physically with sound and gesture) their chosen animal whilst meeting the gaze of another in circle. That person responds by imitating their animal to another in the group and so on.
	Exploding engine
	Participants stand in circle and begin by stamping both feet, beginning slowly and becoming faster and louder. At the same time they make a 'whistling' sound which gets louder and continues until all are out of breath.
Becoming comfortable with touch	*The snake*
	Participants join hands with a person next to them until a long 'snake' is formed. The 'snake' then twists and turns as people move around the room whilst maintaining contact, for example, going under others' linked hands or through legs until a large knot is formed. Participants must try to untangle whilst maintaining joined hands.
	The soft wall
	Participants form a tight circle (the soft wall) and a volunteer stands in the middle with arms by their sides. The volunteer (with closed eyes) allows their body to relax and flop from side to side, being gently 'caught' as the members of the soft wall use their palms to support the volunteer's back. Members of the wall must communicate to ensure that the person in the middle does not fall.

Focus	Suggested exercises
Developing improvisation skills	*What's next?* A facilitator suggests a scene, for example waiting at a bus stop. Participants take turns to join the scene and act a character appropriate to that scene – bin man, old lady, mother pushing a pushchair, etc. *Mini-sketch* Participants are put in groups of three to five and are given a theme, for example, getting out of bed, an arrest, late night on a hospital ward. They are given 20–30 minutes to prepare an improvised sketch to perform to the rest of the group. The sketch may be given a genre – comedy, tragedy, drama, etc.
Building trust	*Follow the leader* Participants are paired and take turns in verbally leading (but not touching) each other around a space. The 'led' person has their eyes closed (as if wearing a blindfold), so is reliant on the leader to alert them to any obstacles, for example chairs, walls and other people. *The bridge* Participants are paired with someone of comparable physical stature. They sit back-to-back with their knees bent. They must then work together to stand simultaneously whilst keeping their backs pressed together.
Enacting emotion	*Being a feeling* Participants are spread around the space and asked to act out an emotion, for example happiness, disgust, anger, grief or joy. They must use their whole body. All participants do this simultaneously, with the facilitator giving instructions such as: How does your face look? Where are you? Who is with you? What can you see? What can you smell?
Responding to direction	*Stop-go* Participants are instructed to walk randomly around a space. The facilitator gives different commands which the participants respond to: 'go'– walk forward, normal pace; 'fast forward'– walk forward quickly; 'reverse'– walk backwards at normal pace; 'stop'– stop walking; 'zig zag'– walk in zig zag pattern. These commands can also be reversed, for example, stop becomes go and go becomes stop. *What's your class?* Participants are instructed to walk randomly around the space in the room. They are asked to adopt a role according to a particular social class or status: 0 would represent someone from the lowest class imaginable and 10, someone from the highest class. They are instructed to adapt their posture, pace and movement according to the class they have selected and to *be* that person. They should then change class (and associated characteristics) as facilitator changes number to 2, 3, 4, 5, etc. Participants are then asked to select a role according to a particular class as described above and to interact with others in the group according to that class. This should be based on gesture, posture and eye contact rather than speech and sound. Afterwards the facilitator asks participants which class they felt most comfortable acting and why. This can be adapted into a scenario where people of different classes have to act out a scene where they interact with each other.

(continued)

Focus	Suggested exercises
Developing observational skills	*The mirror* Participants are paired and instructed to make simple movements and gestures that are mirrored (copied) by the other. Participants then mouth (but don't verbalise) a variety of commands and statements to their partner whilst backing away from each other but maintaining eye contact. The listener/observer has to try to comprehend what is being said and the accompanying emotion which is fed back to their partner. Roles are then reversed and process is repeated.
Developing empathic skills	*Me-picture* Participants work in groups of four. Large sheets of paper, coloured pens and pencils are made available. Each group member draws something to describe themselves. Other group members have to discuss and try to decipher what has been drawn without the 'drawer' verbalising.
Developing voice projection	*Vocal exercises* Participants stand in a circle with shoulders back and legs slightly apart. All repeat vocal sounds spoken clearly (and fairly loudly) by facilitator: 'bappity, beppity, bippoty, boppity, buppity'. This is continued using different consonants: 'cappity, ceppity, cippity, coppity, cuppity', etc. The sounds should be spoken loudly, clearly and quickly and repeated twice each before moving to the next consonant. Participants should ensure that they are breathing deeply from their diaphragm.
Developing breathing control	*Yogic breathing* Participants form a circle, standing straight and tall with legs firmly planted and slightly apart. Shoulders should be rotated backwards and then forwards three times each. Ensure that the shoulders are rolled back and that they are not tense and hunching towards the ears. Stretch arms upwards and reach as high as possible, then repeat, this time standing on tiptoes. Each person focuses on their breathing with their eyes closed, ensuring that the breath comes from the diaphragm rather than the chest. Participants can place their hands on the abdomen to check that they can feel the diaphragm expanding as they take a breath. They should focus on the breath in three parts; as the breath is taken from the diaphragm, as it moves into the chest and as they breath out through the nose or mouth.
Developing movement	*Pass a clap* Participants stand in a circle and 'pass a clap' around it. Each claps as quickly and as loudly as possible and turns to face person next to them as they do so. Facilitator should begin clockwise and switch to anti-clockwise on several occasions to get participants accustomed to attending to cues and direction. *Kung-fu kick* Each participant takes it in turn to simulate a kung-fu 'attack' on another member of the group with whom they make eye contact. Each person mimics an exaggerated kung-fu movement and accompanying sound, for example, 'hiiii-yaaaa'. The person 'attacked' responds by contorting their body and groaning/yelling as if attacked. After recovering, they then choose another member of the group to attack until all have had a turn.

CONCLUSION

This chapter has outlined the utility of acting and drama in mental health education. It is a teaching medium that can address many of the shortcomings of role play and is particularly suited to mental health teaching in its focus on embodiment and emotional experiences. It facilitates the safe exploration of mental distress and can provide an outlet for those working in a stressful environment. I hope that the use of examples and associated resources will provide a structure for others who wish to develop this type of teaching.

RESOURCES

Boal A. *Games for Actors And Non-actors*. 2nd ed. London: Routledge; 2002.

The British Association of Dramatherapists www.badth.org.uk/

National Association for Drama Therapy (USA) www.nadt.org/

The Stanislavski Centre www.stanislavskicentre.org.uk/

ACKNOWLEDGEMENTS

I am indebted to my talented and inspiring acting colleagues Mike Crook, Elaine Grews, Lucy Greaves and Simon Sanchez from whom I learnt many of the exercises and techniques presented. With thanks to my colleague Dr Martin von Fragstein and Dr Stuart Whan.

REFERENCES

1 Shakespeare W. *Hamlet, Prince of Denmark*. Edwards P (editor). Cambridge: Cambridge University Press; 2003. Act 2, Scene 1. p. 155.

2 Parsons T. *The Social System*. New York: Free Press; 1951.

3 Kurtz S, Silverman J, Draper J. *Teaching and Learning Communication Skills in Medicine*. 2nd ed. Oxford: Radcliffe Publishing; 2005.

4 Powley D. The drama of everyday life. In: Powley E, Higson R (editors). *The Arts in Medical Education*. Oxford: Radcliffe Publishing; 2005.

5 Rosenbaum ME, Ferguson KJ, Herwaldt LA. In their own words: presenting the patient's perspective using research-based theatre. *Med Educ*. 2005; **39**(6): 622–31.

6 Case GA, Brauner DJ. Perspective: the doctor as performer: a proposal for change based on a performance studies paradigm. *Acad Med*. 2010; **85**(1): 159–63.

7 Boal A. *The Theatre of the Oppressed*. London: Pluto Press; 1974.

8 Whyman R. The actor's second nature: Stanislavski and William James. *New Theat Q*. 2007; **23**(90): 115–23.

9 Williams T. *A Streetcar Named Desire*. Oxford: Heinemann; 1947.

10 Burton NL. *Psychiatry*. Oxford: Blackwell; 2006.

CHAPTER 12

Music and psychiatry

Neil Nixon

INTRODUCTION

This chapter presents ways of teaching psychiatry through music, not as it ought to be done but as it might be done. The methods and materials described here do not rest on an acknowledged body of literature but have emerged largely through local discussion involving the Division of Psychiatry and School of Music at the University of Nottingham. Through evolution, rather than design, the course has concentrated on post-Renaissance, Western music. I took a more conscious decision to focus on particular individuals, rather than attempt to cover a broad range, or list of cases. This reflects a belief that genuine understanding in psychiatry and music takes time to develop. The principles I have chosen are Robert Schumann (1810–56) and *Peter Grimes* (opera by Benjamin Britten, 1945). Both are brought together through words and music; with Schumann through biography; and in *Grimes* through the libretto. I am deeply indebted to scholarship on Schumann, who lived through severe psychiatric disorder, and the character of Peter Grimes, who acts as a portrayal, but perhaps also a working through, of more complex, liminal areas that dramatise and problematise for us what psychiatry is and what it has been.

WHY STUDY MUSIC AND PSYCHIATRY?

How might music genuinely add to an understanding of psychiatry? Immediately, one could answer that music helps us embed our study within wider cultural understandings and for a medical world often criticised for being too inward looking this might be good enough. But there is an equally powerful answer within music itself, which holds the promise of bringing normally silent thoughts and feelings to the surface of things, giving psychology presence. And whilst we can never hope to demonstrate psychological processes in the way that a surgeon can show physical processes, we can certainly identify mental phenomena in music. This may be because a composer explicitly intended to communicate personal, lived experience this way, as with Schönberg's conscious recreation of his cardiac pain in the String Trio, Op. 45, completed shortly after a massive myocardial infarction. Alternatively, it may be through music drama, such as an opera in which someone appears to ignore darker thematic intimations, responding selectively to brighter music, in an attempt to deny unpleasant reality. Or through people coming together in sustained dissonance, a psychologically unpleasant phenomenon, creating the feeling that whatever may be said more consciously, at a deeper level there may be uncomfortable disagreement. In these ways music may lend substance to psychology and help students grasp what is otherwise often missed.

Approaching these phenomena of experience, not simply within the narrow confines of medicine but within the depths of our shared culture, brings us to basic questions about the nature of difference, rather than simply assuming this as a starting point. These questions of difference, often central to medical students' conception of psychiatry and 'psychiatric patients', tend to remain implicit, unchallenged or even reinforced through psychiatric placements and into medical careers. But here we can question why *Grimes*, Britten and Schumann might ever have been considered to suffer 'psychiatric problems' and how such different stories could be incorporated under a common rubric. We can question the persistence of such general, homogenous terms to denote people; how these terms influence our understanding of important aspects of identity, including work; and how they may change the way that people are treated. Does music identified with 'madness', such as Schumann's late work, help us understand something central to our shared humanity or is it the tainted work of illness, better buried or destroyed?

Through works like *Peter Grimes* we can not only identify difference musically and psychologically but also explore ways of understanding other people, through dramatised perspectives. In this we quickly find that students' reflections on ways of seeing other people become personal and ideas of privileged positions, outside of humanity, from which to make complex judgments are experientially challenged. The drama and music in *Peter Grimes* give a powerful focus for exploring the limits of the positions we take as doctors and human beings.

Through all of this students are directed to questions of difference, worth and perspective that often run unseen within psychiatry and medicine, only occasionally bubbling to the surface. These questions come to the surface when a medical student asks to talk with her teacher after a lecture on obsessive-compulsive disorder, finally able to say after years that she has been suffering in this way and suddenly the question arises, 'am I mad?' in other words 'am I now the observer or the observed?' and more deeply 'am I still worthwhile?' They come to the surface when a supportive doctor becomes, too late, aware that her patient has abused a child and finds a critical community asking how this could have happened, 'how could she have seen things that way?' It is at these points that we see medicine most clearly, not simply as a laboratory science but as a human science. It is precisely at these points that we might help our future doctors and their patients by exploring 'madness' not as alien to life but as part of our shared humanity.

INTRODUCING MEDICAL STUDENTS TO WORKING WITH MUSIC

Not all medical students have a background in music and so we begin by trying to make people feel comfortable working with it. We have chosen to do this by using already shared experience in science, and embedding Western tonal music in its physicality, physiology and brain function. This understanding of the physical importance of music, formed part of Daniel Barenboim's 2006 Reith Lectures[1] and in our introduction makes use of recent advances in brain imaging, mainly functional magnetic resonance imaging (fMRI), and brain electrophysiology, principally event-related potentials (ERPs). We start by playing one note on the piano and follow sound within the room – through the standing wav, the atmosphere, the outer and inner ear, into phase-locked, tonotopic transmission through the nervous system.

We demonstrate this physicality of music, transmitted through us without boundaries in normal physiology and linking us absolutely with our environment. We cover recent experiments in brain function during the processing of regular versus irregular chord progressions; during dissonance versus consonance; and semantic priming in language and music.[2,3,4] There is no space here to explore this research in any detail but it introduces important musical concepts alongside evidence that, at least within Western culture, even people with little formal background in music can pick up quite subtle aspects of musical structure and meaning. Further, it provides evidence that the functional brain activity underlying musical understanding can occur without full conscious awareness, even when music appears unimportant within a situation, suggesting that we may not always be fully aware of the extent of our musical abilities. Students can experience this by identifying the point at which short piano phrases 'sound irregular'. We use phrases that start off with standard tonic-dominant-tonic progressions followed by phrases with irregular endings (using Neapolitan chords). Although none of the students has been able to articulate the technical aspects of this change, they have without fail identified the musical irregularity at a basic level; a level at which they are apparently all musicians whether they know it or not.

Another way to involve students in music is to help one of them play a highly dissonant chord, such as a tritone, next to a consonant interval. The experience of dissonance, usually described as unpleasant, can be discussed in terms of its importance to music and then linked to work showing that permanently dissonant music increases brain activity in a network including the amygdala more often stimulated in neuropsychology through presentation of frightening pictures and in neuropsychiatry being closely linked to trauma, anxiety and clinical depression.[5]

LIVED EXPERIENCE: ROBERT SCHUMANN (1810–56)

Whilst we do not know the exact nature of Robert Schumann's psychiatric problems, we can be confident that he suffered very severe psychiatric disorder. We know that he continued to compose music during a period of psychosis and that those closest to him were painfully aware of this, destroying or withholding much of his late work. Although now over 150 years old, we have impressive contemporaneous documentation and intimate music that supports and breathes life into this story, bringing us to the nature and social understanding of 'madness'.

We begin with a traditional biographical narrative, accompanied by some shorter pieces for the piano, such as Carnival, Op. 9, Nos 24 and 25, and sections of longer works, such as the Fantasy (Grand Sonata) in C, Op. 17, that help to support the story and show some aspects of Schumann's early musical style. The two pieces from Carnival, entitled Eusebius and Florestan, are used to illustrate different states of being that Schumann identified in himself, as the introspective Eusebius or more flamboyant Florestan. The Fantasy, Op. 17, illustrates Schumann's mental state within a period of enforced separation from the woman he loved and thought he was losing, but who in fact later became his wife, Clara. This latter piece, written in the key of C (possibly for Clara) contains quite conscious musical quotes of Beethoven's 'An die ferne Geliebte' (To the distant beloved). As Schumann later wrote to Clara, 'you can only understand the Fantasy if you imagine yourself in the unhappy summer of 1836, when I gave you up'.[6] For Schumann then, all three of these pieces were deeply personal accounts reflecting different psychological states.

We use piano music in the earlier part of this biography, partly to enhance comparison with music written during Schumann's evolving, severe psychosis of 1854. By that time, the occasional experience of hearing a single tone A, not heard by other people, had developed through intervals to fully orchestrated music that was initially 'more wonderful than ever one hears on earth', but later the cause of dreadful suffering associated with clear accounts of visual hallucinations, complex auditory hallucinations, evolving delusions and possible cognitive impairment.[7] Within this state Schumann is documented as having said that either an angel, or the then-dead Franz Schubert, dictated a musical theme to him. This theme is in fact readily identifiable in the second movement of Schumann's violin concerto of 1853 but apparently unaware he had used it before, perhaps experiencing it now as a complex auditory hallucination, he wrote out the simple E flat major theme with five variations, published as the Ghost Variations (WoO 24). Within hours of completing a first draft, Schumann made a violent attempt at suicide, only narrowly failing. Days later, he dedicated the final manuscript of this final piano work to Clara who had by that time left their home on the advice of a physician fearful of her safety.[8] Within weeks Robert Schumann admitted himself voluntarily to Endenich asylum where he died just over two years later.

We listen to the E flat theme and variations in the context of this story and the earlier piano music. The theme is calm, perhaps resignedly melancholic and according to one student, 'much too calm for someone who was about to attempt suicide'. In fact, sudden calmness, following more agitated distress, often prefigures completed suicide in a way that can mislead both loved ones and professionals. The variations, composed during Schumann's psychosis, retain the introspective feeling of the theme without the expansive development seen in earlier work, such as Op. 17. They feel denser, less gentle, less clearly structured and more dissonant than the E flat theme. The first variation creates frequent dissonance through repeated minor seconds, with an intricate internal melody tightly caught between inner and outer phrasing that has the overall effect of blurring the clarity of the theme without greatly developing it. The third variation threatens to become more flamboyant but never fully develops. There is very little in this work that suggests a manic phase of bipolar disorder. Perhaps instead there is a disintegrated, melancholy awareness of what was beginning.

We then present a medical/psychiatric account of Schumann from the point of his admission to Endenich. This is a way of using the available phenomenology to arrive at potential medical formulations. It is also a way of comparing the perspectives of biographical and medical narratives. We discuss aspects of Schumann's family history, medical history and personality that may have made him vulnerable to psychiatric disorder and consider a wide range of main and subsidiary diagnoses, including organic illness (such as general paralysis of the insane), bipolar disorder and recurrent depressive disorder. The point of this is not to establish 'the truth' of Schumann's psychiatric disorder but instead to debate the possibilities.

We finally consider how this illness affected the perception of Schumann's late work. The Ghost Variations of 1854 and violin concerto of 1853 were both deliberately held back from publication until the late 1930s. Although the concerto is now considered an important part of the repertoire, Joseph Joachim for whom it was written, never played it in public. Other works from this time, including a set of romances for cello, appear to have been deliberately destroyed. Why was this immediate reaction so different to the current opinion of many violinists who see the concerto as an important work? What might have caused this reaction and how should we respond to work associated with mental illness? If there is a chance that the mental state evoked is not introspection, flamboyance or loss but instead psychosis, should we then keep this work away from others, perhaps even destroy it? Students have been able to see how intimate Schumann's music was to Clara and can understand the grief, fear and love involved in her reaction to her husband. They have been equally grateful for the chance to listen to his late music that may, with all its idiosyncrasies, tell us something important about a very human state.

PORTRAYED EXPERIENCE: OPERA AND *PETER GRIMES*

Even within the relatively narrow scope of post-Renaissance Western music there is rich opportunity to explore the portrayal of madness. For several reasons we have decided to focus on opera. To begin with, opera combines an explicit drama with a musical accompaniment that is often intended to convey psychological meaning. The explicit presence of normally silent psychological worlds alongside public drama presents an extra dimension, often missed or neglected in life, that can bring mental states to shared attention.

In addition to this basic structure, opera has shown an apparent interest in 'madness' through the 'mad scene' and in part through the high incidence of suicide. This interest, which reached a peak in early Romantic opera (1800–50), coincided with a generally greater public interest in psychiatry in Europe. In England, a rich combination of high profile legal cases, such as those involving James Hadfield and

Daniel McNaughton, together with the suffering of prominent figures, including King George III, had led to intense debate about the organisation and treatment of 'insanity'. This argument resolved partly through the English County Asylum Acts (1808, 1845), which were in keeping with the French *loi sur les aliénés* (1838), and the drive evident through much of Europe to contain and treat psychiatric disorder in asylums run by physicians. These important early steps in the medicalisation of 'lunacy' were accompanied by the withdrawal of religion, and an intensification of interest through opera in the context and nature of 'madness'.

Although there is a coincidence of interest here, between early Romantic opera and the public medicalisation of 'madness', there are also clear points of departure that we needed to think through before using opera as a device for teaching psychiatry. For instance, 'madness' often appeared to physicians in the nineteenth century as of likely organic or simply indeterminate cause, whereas in opera, as Jones suggests, it is almost always an understandable phenomenon, emerging from the interpersonal narrative.[9] Secondly, even within the legal sanctions of the nineteenth century there is frequent evidence of failed suicide and deliberate self-harm, evident in both court and asylum records but in opera, as Feggetter points out, almost any self-harm results in completed suicide.[10] In opera then, 'madness' tends to emerge in an understandable way, followed by a quick end, as one might expect of a dramatic device intended principally to serve the narrative and music. In life, as we teach through Robert Schumann, one of the greatest early Romantic composers, even violent suicide attempts could fail, leaving 'madness' unresolved, protracted and frighteningly dissociated from any understandable precursors.

With these caveats, we have used early 'mad scenes' to explore psychological states and the portrayal of difference. Using probably the most famous of all 'mad scenes' in *Lucia di Lammermoor* (Donizetti, Naples, 1835) we have looked at trauma, dissociation and psychosis. The music gives Lucia's mental state a powerful reality alongside the drama of the 'mad scene', perhaps enhanced by Donizetti's use of flutes signaling to early nineteenth-century audiences that they were being directed to Lucia's internal state. Alongside her separate struggle, heard through the orchestra, we see vividly in most productions the reactions of those around Lucia, including fear, perplexity and disgust. We have used a number of other early Romantic operas in this way, including *Macbeth* (Verdi, Florence, 1849), but have focused on a much later opera by Benjamin Britten that highlights alienation within a community that resolves in the 'madness' and suicide of its central protagonist, Peter Grimes.

Peter Grimes was written by the pacifist Britten during the Second World War and premiered by Sadler's Wells Opera in July 1945, with Peter Pears, Britten's life-long partner in the lead role. The beginnings of this opera were deeply personal for Britten, who in the California of 1941, came across a work by George Crabbe, set in his native Suffolk that produced 'a longing for the realities of that grim and exciting seacoast around Aldeburgh'.[11] This nostalgia must have been tempered by an uncomfortable awareness that, as a pacifist and homosexual, the composer would be an outsider in wartime England. As written by Crabbe, Grimes is a sadistically violent man who, 'knew not justice' and ended his life telling 'a madman's tale' in a parish bed.[12] In

Britten's work, the outsider becomes much more ambiguous. Whereas Crabbe's Grimes takes pleasure in violence, Britten's character suffers through the impulsive or accidental violence he causes as part of his personality and central drive to overcome through work. Britten then, returning to his longed-for England in 1941, with his own ambitions, told a much softer tale of the outsider, with empathy but perhaps also with the sympathy he hoped to receive himself. *Peter Grimes* delivers not only an inspired account of the nature of the outsider, topographically and psychologically, but expresses a realism that was deep within Britten himself.

The rich promise of this opera in teaching psychiatry comes partly from this proximity of reality and drama. The World Health Organization assumed responsibility for the International Classification of Diseases (ICD) with its sixth edition in 1948 and included homosexuality in this and subsequent revisions until it was removed from the ninth revision, published in 1977. The American Psychiatric Association followed this trend of viewing homosexuality as a psychiatric disorder, backed up by US surveys showing that even by 1974 over 70% of people felt 'sex acts between two persons of the same sex . . . were always wrong even if they love each other'.[13] Britten died in 1976. Within his lifetime men were not only 'diagnosed' with homosexuality, they could be coerced into anti-androgen treatment even if they had served their country with distinction, as in the case of Alan Turing, who carried out vital work for the allies during the Second World War, before suffering imposed 'treatment for homosexuality', which was followed by his eventual suicide in 1954. So any fear that Britten may have had as an outsider was well founded.

In *Peter Grimes* the opera, the outsider is from the outset depicted in his words and music as cut off, both from himself and from the community. The prologue of the opera shows Grimes defending himself in court following the death of an apprentice boy in his care. Although the inquest settles on death in 'accidental circumstances', Peter Grimes' words fail to convince the Suffolk community of his innocence. Musically, the terse a cappella of the examining magistrate contrasts with the orchestral strings accompanying Grimes' statements, suggesting an innocence that at least Grimes is convinced of himself. The frustration of not being able to communicate this and of not being believed is deeply felt by Grimes, who 'cannot show, let alone prove his tenderness . . . except through the music which, alas, the people on the stage don't hear'.[14] From this early point then the outsider is set up as someone who at least believes in what he says but cannot convey this to others.

The cohesion of the community, against natural storms and against Peter Grimes, is reinforced through its shared music, harmonised at critical points in B flat or E flat, creating dissonant minor seconds during references to Grimes, in A, E or B.[15] This effect is heard from the opera's opening in B flat, suddenly jarring with the very first words, which fall on A, 'Peter Grimes . . . Peter Grimes . . . Peter Grimes'. Because A is one semitone from B flat we hear a dissonant minor second with this first mention of the name 'Peter Grimes', immediately setting him apart as an undermining, discordant influence within society. When, in Act 1, scene 1, Grimes enters in E flat himself, the community has been singing in calm unison for almost 8 minutes around the key of A, so his entrance creates immediate, extreme dissonance, through the unpleasant effect of a tritone, 'the Devil's interval'.[16] This musical dissonance, associated with the actual and psychological presence of Grimes in his community, continues from the first mention of his name, almost without break, until the tension can no longer be contained and Grimes becomes the object of a manhunt.

Grimes is offered one break within all of this, through the widowed schoolmistress Ellen Orford, who takes a much more sympathetic approach and through this manages to bring him lyrically and musically to her. This brief connection comes in the wake of the trial that has left Grimes bitter and persecuted; a mood that he expresses in F minor. Ellen is with him physically but is psychologically in a different, more hopeful world, expressed both in her words and in her music in E major. Towards the end of what might loosely be termed an aria, Grimes is won through Ellen's sympathy, joining her musically, lyrically and psychologically in E major. It is important to our teaching that this brief psychological connection comes through Ellen sympathetically encouraging Grimes to join her hope rather than trying to enter and understand his bleaker world through empathy. Aspects of Grimes' world may be seen in this brief union, through the repeated, shared minor 9ths, a dissonant interval of 13 semitones associated with Grimes' bleak isolation throughout the rest of the opera. But these minor 9ths also emphasise the superficial, fragile nature of the link between Grimes and Ellen and their relationship, which is characterised by phantasy.

The cost of Ellen's sympathy and her lack of real understanding, comes in her helping Grimes to obtain another apprentice boy from the local workhouse, despite the misgivings of the wider community who are more overtly concerned with the risk Grimes might pose. Grimes uses this second apprentice in an attempt to prove himself to the local community and as the drama plays out, the boy, who is given no voice in the opera, is at the very least severely neglected by Grimes. Ellen clearly has intimations of this abuse in the early music of Act 2, scene 1, but chooses to ignore these darker themes in favour of brighter music from a nearby church. When she finally notices a bruise on the apprentice, her denial is critically challenged. Her efforts to gently explore what has happened to the boy trigger Grimes' sense of persecution. He hits her impulsively, and realises he has lost her. As his phantasies become untenable in an increasingly constrained reality, the community launches a manhunt and Grimes responds by driving his apprentice boy even harder, literally over a cliff, where the boy falls and dies.

Grimes, now responsible for the deaths of two young boys, decompensates during what is often referred to as his 'mad scene' but might otherwise be construed as a psychological crisis in which he is caught between an intense fear of remaining and his basic attachment to this place, his Suffolk home. He has no one now to turn to and so works through his crisis in soliloquy, appearing perplexed and remorseful during fragmentary renderings of the deaths he is responsible for amidst thoughts and fears for his future. Philip Brett points out that musically, in this mental state, the minor seconds given to Grimes are in fact an inversion of the community's motif in the courtroom at the beginning of the opera.[17] Grimes has musically turned the anger and hatred of the community in on himself, just as his derogatory repetition of his own name 'Grimes . . . Grimes' does this linguistically. With his defenses down, in crisis, Grimes is offered a way out of his dilemma and submits to the suggestion that he might kill himself at sea. The opera finishes with the community still perversely connected to Grimes, watching his ship sink, whilst we presume Grimes is drowning.

We work through this, as a teaching device, by asking students to take different perspectives to the main protagonist, including those of Ellen Orford and the community. The counterpoise is between sympathetic support and a more alienating criticism; between Ellen's initial success in making some connection, however fragile, as against what people have seen as her denial of the more abusive aspects of Grimes; between the thoughtless alienation of the community and perhaps its more realistic understanding of risk. Within these perspectives, we also ask a student to consider Grimes' personality and how this affects the dynamic he is central to. The dramatisation of these approaches to the troubled protagonist opens up a dilemma often felt by doctors but poorly explored; namely where to place oneself between sympathy for an individual and wider public protection. It also allows the introduction of the alternative approach of empathy, advocated in psychiatry since Karl Jaspers, as a way to understand the phenomena of human experience in other people; to get at the undercurrent suggested by the music. And we can feel in Grimes' bleak music how difficult true empathy can be, how uncomfortable it can be to enter a world like this, why it might more easily be avoided and at what cost.

The question of why Britten in particular wrote this opera opens a door on the history of psychiatry. The idea that Britten, like Schumann, could potentially have been 'diagnosed' with a psychiatric disorder by his contemporaries is usually surprising to medical students. He no longer fits the broad category of 'madness' in the way that Schumann does, but even if Britten is a long way from current conceptions of psychiatric disorder, we can still point to the relatively recent listing of 'homosexuality' by the World Health Organization in its classification of diseases. This historical contingency of difference can be set next to its continuing importance for group psychology. Students can readily see how, in *Peter Grimes*, 'members' of the community receive relative protection through their group identity, despite pursuing unhealthy individual interests, such as laudanum addiction. They can see the outsider dramatised as a common, distracting focus for general discontents. They can experience the corrosive power of stigma as well as its binding force, operating within the group and the word 'madness'. The continual stream of contemporary cases of brutal social out-grouping add disturbing relevance to this story and always seem to update Peter Pears' comment from 1946 that, 'There are plenty of Grimeses around still, I think!'[18]

WHAT DO WE NEED TO STUDY THIS AREA?

The key elements for teaching music with psychiatry are time and space. My experience suggests that the teaching only works well when we take time to fully listen to the complete works we are focusing on. Because the opera *Peter Grimes* can take up to three hours, the students are asked to listen to it between seminars and we then review key scenes together.

With regard to space I am deeply indebted to the School of Music at the University of Nottingham for making their resources available, thereby allowing us to play music comfortably, through recordings or the piano. I am also grateful to the clinicians and academic staff from psychiatry and music who have joined the teaching with enthusiasm and great insight.

CONCLUDING REMARKS

At the beginning of this, I had already been in medical education as a lecturer and a clinician for some time. Through my interest, I often incorporated elements of wider culture into lectures, without ever feeling I had come close to using its full potential. For me, this new course was above all an opportunity to explore whether music could be effectively used to teach aspects of psychiatry.

The experience and feedback of the last few years has been much more positive than I ever imagined. Students have engaged in discussions around the basic human aspects of our science and our role as doctors in ways that are rarely achieved in more traditional teaching. Hearing the music of Schumann and Britten alongside their stories has seemed to create an atmosphere allowing us more easily into discussions that are otherwise often stilted, neglected or missed.

As one comes closer to these works they feel less easily divided into 'lived' and 'portrayed' experience. One becomes more aware of them as personal expressions, unexpectedly connecting Schumann, Britten and Grimes in their very human problems. Through them we are connected to 'otherness' and made aware of reactions to it, including our own. We are involved in the problem that has always been present in attempts to stand apart from the world, even through calling parts of it 'madness', and in the end remain as doctors and human beings connected to it for good or ill.

REFERENCES

1　Barenboim D. Lecture 1: In the beginning was sound. BBC Reith Lectures; 2006. Available at: www.bbc.co.uk/radio4/reith2006/lecture1.shtml (accessed 15 May 2010).

2　Koelsch S. Neural substrates of processing syntax and semantics in music. *Curr Opin Neurol.* 2005; **15**: 1–6.

3　Koelsch S, Fritz T, von Cramon DY, *et al.* Investigating emotion with music: an fMRI study. *Hum Brain Mapp.* 2006; **27**: 239–50.

4　Koelsch S, Kasper E, Sammler D, *et al.* Music, language, and meaning: brain signatures of semantic processing. *Nat Neurosci.* 2004; **7**: 302–7.

5　Koelsch S, Fritz T, *et al.* Investigating emotion with music: an fMRI study. *Hum Brain Mapp.* 2006; **27**: 239–50.

6　Worthen J. *Robert Schumann: life and death of a musician.* New Haven and London: Yale University Press; 2007.

7   Ibid.

8   Seiffert W-D. *Schumann Variations on a Theme (Ghost Variations)*. Munich: Urtext G Henle Verlag; 1995.

9   Jones M. The psychiatry of opera. *Psychiatr Bull.* 1990; **14**: 556–7.

10 Feggetter G. Suicide in opera: *Lucia di Lammermoor. Br J of Psychiatr.* 1980; **136**: 552–7.

11 Britten B. Introduction. In: Banks P (editor). *The Making of Peter Grimes*. Woodbridge: The Boydell Press; 2000. pp. 1–3.

12 Crabbe G. *The Borough: a poem in twenty-four letters*. London: J Hatchard; 1810.

13 Levitt EE, Klassen AD. Public attitudes toward homosexuality: part of the 1970 national survey by the Institute for Sex Research. *J Homosex.* 1974; **1**(1): 29–43.

14 Keller H. 'Peter Grimes': the story, the music not excluded. In: Brett P (editor). *Peter Grimes*. Cambridge: Cambridge University Press; 1983. pp. 105–20.

15 Brett P. Britten and Grimes. In: Brett P (editor). *Peter Grimes*. Cambridge: Cambridge University Press; 1983. pp. 180–9.

16 Metropolitan Opera Guild. *Met School Membership Program:* Peter Grimes. Opera News: The Metropolitan Opera Guild Inc; 1999.

17 Brett P (editor). *Peter Grimes*. Cambridge: Cambridge University Press; 1983.

18 Pears P. Neither a hero nor a villain. In: Brett P (editor). *Peter Grimes*. Cambridge: Cambridge University Press; 1983. pp. 150–2.

CHAPTER 13

What can we learn from blues music?

David Dodwell

Music is the 'aesthetic mean between chaotic irregularity and monotonous regularity'.[1]

INTRODUCTION

I initially gave a workshop on this subject based on my personal interest in blues music and as a challenge to explore its educational potential. My approach is consciously non-linear, exploratory, and derived from humanities values rather than 'hard' science values. I am writing as a psychiatrist with an amateur's love of the blues: I am neither a musicologist nor a music therapist.

This chapter will describe some aspects of blues music specifically; discuss some aspects of music generally; and briefly refer to how an interactive workshop can make use of this information. I shall consider learning points throughout the text.

Blues music

Blues music provides a relatively contained art form linked to specific social contexts. It probably emerged around 1900: and has been in intermittent decline since around 1960 (particularly within its root social group).[2] It therefore occupies a space in recent, recorded history, although its social context means that records (in both senses) are far from complete.

'The blues' can also refer to low mood. There is clearly an overlap between having the blues and playing the blues, but not all blues music is sad.[3] Many of the messages I wish to convey could be portrayed using other musical forms.

SOCIAL HISTORY OF THE BLUES

Human beings are produced from a combination of genetic material from each parent developing in and interacting with the environment they inhabit. Blues is similarly a product of material from different sources, which has combined and developed in an environmental context. Black people were transported from West

Africa as slaves to work in the southern United States (US), where they were exposed to different instruments, different rules (e.g. a ban on using drums) and other musical traditions. Of course, other new musical forms developed from migrations, both of white non-slaves (e.g. Cajun, bluegrass), and from importation of black slaves to other areas of the New World (e.g. Samba, Salsa, Son, Ska).

Those enslaved typically dwelt in inland Africa and were initially caught by black coastal slave-traders who sold them on. The conditions in which these human goods were warehoused before and during transport were appalling and there was a high death rate during the voyage from Africa to America. The various steps in the process tended to destroy the normal social links of family and tribe or clan. Treatment in the US no doubt varied from owner to owner but could often be brutal. Killing a slave was not considered criminal as long as a substitute, or money to buy one, was provided. Despite the harsh life and frequent early death, the desire to run away was defined as a mental illness – drapetomania.[4] Indifference to African-American life continued for longer than one might expect, for example the Tuskagee Syphilis experiment was not terminated until 1972 and was not apologised for until 1997.[5]

Slaves were converted to Christianity, although some traditional beliefs and practices continued alongside or in an assimilated form. Understandably, Biblical passages concerning the enslavement and deportation/exile of the Jews (to Egypt or Babylon) held a certain resonance.

Apart from casual brutality, rape and killing, slave life had a number of more regular constraints. There could be limits on dancing and/or music which might make church the only opportunity for such activities; on the other hand, it is said a ban on slaves using drums in most parts of the US led to a secularisation of music due to the loss of traditional religious rituals.[6] It has been suggested that white men took no notice of sung lyrics, so words that could not be spoken could be voiced in song.[7]

Although slavery officially ended with the conclusion of the civil war in 1865, the southern agricultural system continued using the 'sharecropper' system, which became a form of serfdom due to the monopolies held by the white landowners (there is evidence that black tenants were preferred because they were easier to oppress than white tenants).[8] Civil rights were rapidly eroded, violence by whites against blacks was largely ignored, and segregation continued, perpetuating for decades conditions almost as disadvantageous and damaging as slavery. Agriculture tended to rely on undiversified single crops, such as cotton or tobacco, which made it vulnerable to disease (e.g. the cotton boll weevil) or market failure. The geography held a risk of flooding (broad flat lands with banked irrigation channels – levees – and the huge Mississippi river) and over-cultivation led to the dust-bowl phenomenon.

The development of road and rail transport made it increasingly possible to escape a harsh, exploitative rural setting. There was a tendency to move into cities. In particular, there was a tendency to move to northern industrial cities, such as Chicago and Detroit, which were seen as likely to offer improved employment prospects, more money and less racist persecution.

In addition to their individual heritage, African-American people have been exposed to the same influences as other inhabitants of the US. The twentieth century has seen the growth of capitalism, advertising, organised crime, failed attempts to control substance abuse, the Depression, two World Wars and the 'Cold War'.

MUSICAL ROOTS OF THE BLUES

We presume that slaves brought with them their local music as memories. It is unlikely that they would have imported instruments but they would have known how to make them. After arrival they would have been exposed to church music and to European instruments. Some would have been taught to play European music for their masters to dance to or be entertained by (a black band could have different repertoires for white or coloured audiences).[9] It is said that the end of the civil war led to demobilisation of military bands and selling of military band instruments which influenced the development of New Orleans jazz. A little-played type of traditional music, 'fife and drum', particularly derives from traditional rather than European instruments. There were a few traditional narrative ballads for example, 'Stag O'Lee' – about a murderer), and 'John Henry' – about a railworker competing with mechanisation.

Singing without instruments continues in the work song tradition. Singing had a value in coordinating actions which were important in some activities (for example two men alternately chopping a tree with their axe) in protecting slower workers from being singled out, and was used to slow down the work rate without the boss' awareness: it continued in prison work gangs until desegregation.[10] The Georgia Sea Islanders also continued a tradition of a cappella singing accompanied by hand claps, some of which appeared to be based on non-Christian West African religious ceremonies.[11] Even speech rhythms are relevant, as is apparent from recordings of sermons.[12] These origins and influences are summarised in Box 13.1.

BOX 13.1 Blues: origins and influences

Speech rhythms
- West African music
  - songs
  - instruments
  - dances
- European church/religious music
- European folk/entertainment music
- European instruments
  - church
  - folk
  - military
  - 'classical'/orchestral
- African-American church music
- African-American work song

Differentiation of blues

From these social and musical origins, a number of types of music evolved in the southern US black communities. The most consistent distinction has been between religious and profane music. Although many blues musicians trace their musical careers back to singing in church, blues was often described as 'the devil's music'. Within secular music, there was initially a broad overlap between blues and jazz, although these strands tended to diverge over time. Ragtime tended to be distinct: highly structured and composed. As noted above, the work song tradition also continued.

What is blues music?

Blues music is hard to define categorically: what follows is a series of generalisations (musical terms are summarised in Box 13.2). Historically, it grew out of the African-American communities of the southern states. Rhythmically, it is usually 4/4 time with strong, regular rhythms supplemented by syncopation and off-beat contrasts. Melodically, it uses a scale which is a hybrid between traditional pentatonic (four note) and European diatonic (seven note), in which the third and seventh notes (blue notes) are prone to be altered from a European 'major' scale by flattening to the minor, by trilling, or by 'bending' into an intermediate note outside the chromatic scale. Song lines often start relatively high and end low.[13] However, other notes can be altered, particularly the fifth, and glissando is common. Harmonically, there is usually a limited, simple structure. Of these three musical elements, one can argue that in European 'classical' music harmony is the most important, followed by melody, and rhythm is unimportant; in Asian music melody is the most important, followed by rhythm, with harmony unimportant; in Africa, rhythm is predominant, and harmony unimportant. In blues, rhythm is perhaps the basis, but all three elements are more equal and none is sophisticated. One vital element in blues is the feeling it conveys, sometimes called 'soul': the importance of soul has been well described by Lorca in a lecture on the cognate concept in Spanish flamenco music of 'duende' – spirit (originally a supernatural spirit akin to the Ancient Greek chthonic daimon).[14,15]

The most common (but not the only) song format is the '12-bar' blues – three musical lines of four bars each and two lines of verse: the first line of verse is sung twice.

BOX 13.2 Some musical terms

Rhythm:	beat
Melody:	sequence of notes, tune
Harmony:	relationship between two or more notes played at the same time
4/4:	standard notation indicating four beats to the bar
Bar:	short, recurring unit of musical time and rhythm
Syncopation:	unexpected or off-beat stress
Scale:	series of accepted notes for constructing melody and harmony

Pentatonic:	five-note scale
Diatonic:	seven-note scale used using selected notes from the Western chromatic scale
Chromatic:	established compromise of 12 notes used in West European classical music, from which scales are selected
Glissando:	sliding from one note to another
Antiphony:	interaction between two individuals or groups – sometimes called 'call and response'

Blues evolved in a non-literate society and therefore belongs to the oral tradition. This distinction is not always well known (for a summary *see* Table 13.1). Performances typically involve a series of building blocks, some of which may carry a narrative and some of which are non-specific fillers, as well as an accepted style and 'vocabulary'. The exact order in which the ingredients are used and the size and shape of the resulting structure varies each time. Personal authorship and innovation are not innately praiseworthy. The values are of familiarity, mirroring and comfort – more like a silver wedding than a first date. The performance may have one co-performer (antiphonist) or a chorus, and the audience may act as a chorus with interjections, repetitions or refrain. Work songs provide a good example: the song leader, singing a solo, is followed by a chorus repeating the line or providing its complement. The effect is inclusive and participatory, partly because it is based on and reaffirms a shared cultural heritage. The mutual interplay was sufficient to cause disquiet to the leader of Georgia Sea Islands singers when performing outside their cultural territory: 'singing in front of these people might change what we do, because of what they do'.[16]

TABLE 13.1 Oral versus literary traditions (from Dodwell)[17]

	Oral	Literary
Authorship	Stewardship	Unique
Audience	Participates	Receives
Sequence	Non-linear	Linear
Novelty	Atavistic	Innovative
Elements	Formulaic	Original
Performances	Extempore	Fixed
Perceived as	Backward	Advanced

Any repeated tale has the risk of becoming stale. The flexibility and interactivity of the oral tradition helped to overcome this, although retaining the 'soul' must remain an essential skill for the performer. Raw authenticity is described by Holiday: 'The blues to me is like being very sad, very sick, going to church, being very happy. There's two kinds of blues: happy blues and sad blues. Anything I do sing is part of my life'.[18]

Varieties of blues

Although the blues has had a relatively short history, there are many varieties as well as grey areas on the periphery. Some of the key parameters are rural versus urban, place, and time. For a representative range of performers *see* Table 13.2.

Biographical data[19]

Rural players tend to rely on more portable instruments and playing alone or in small numbers. They are more likely to have an idiosyncratic style (e.g. Skip James) – John Lee Hooker might well be classed in this way, although residing in Detroit for many years. Urban players have more opportunity to use a wider range of instruments, to play in larger bands, and to be exposed to a greater variety of musical styles.

Defining blues by place is problematic because many musicians are itinerant as part of their work and because of the role of migration in US history. Different types of blues and related music probably originated in different areas of the US, but the heartland seems to be the area round the southern Mississippi River. We know most about blues styles from recordings, which mainly occurred in urban settings. Distinct styles evolved in Chicago, New Orleans and the West Coast. Rural Louisiana evolved its own hybrid, Zydeco, influenced by different instruments (especially piano accordion) and the local French heritage.

Cross-cutting the geographical spread is the temporal evolution, influenced by fashion and technology. Technological variations included changes in instruments and the impacts of amplification and electrification. Fashions were determined by an interaction of musician and audience, so phases of migration could change a local style. There was a clear change in style in recorded Chicago blues from before and after World War II, coinciding with considerable migration. Muddy Waters (McKinley Morganfield) became one of the leading exponents and band leaders of post-war Chicago blues. He was first recorded in 1941 in a rural Mississippi setting by a travelling musicologist from the Library of Congress, Alan Lomax. By 1947 he was being recorded in Chicago, initially with piano and bass, and with a strong rural Mississippi sound.[20] This sound evolved as he added drums, amplified his guitar, and developed a more polished expression.[21,22] No doubt his target audience consisted of migrants from rural areas who were becoming more urbanised. By 1960, this black audience was switching to even more urbane soul music; Muddy Waters recorded at the 1960 Newport Jazz Festival and eventually his audience became white Europeans, with further changes in style to appeal to his new market.

What are blues songs about?

Just as there are elements whose presence or absence act as markers of blues music, there are certain themes that have characteristic presence or absence in blues song lyrics (*see* Box 13.3).

TABLE 13.2 A few blues names

Name	Born–Died	Recording	Birth place	Style	Example	Instruments
Bessie Smith	1894(?)–1937	1923–33	Chattanooga, TN	'Classic'	St Louis Blues	vcl (with band)
Nehemiah 'Skip' James	1902–69	1931; 1964–67	Bentonia, MI	Bentonia	Catfish Blues; I'm So Glad	vcl + ac gtr or pno
Fred McDowell	1904–72	1959–71	Rossville, TN	Mississippi	Louise	vcl + el gtr
Tampa Red[1]	1904–81	1928–60	Smithfield, GA	Pre-war urban	It Hurts Me Too	vcl + gtr (+ gtr/pno/band)
Big Maceo[2]	1905–53	1940s	Atlanta, GA	Urban	Worried Life	pno + vcl (+ gtr/band)
Louis Jordan	1908–75	1930s–70s	Brinkley, AR	Jazz/R&B	Caldonia	vcl + sax (with band)
'T-Bone' Walker	1910–75	1929; 1942–69	Linden, TX	Jazz	Stormy Monday	vcl + el gtr (with band)
Howlin' Wolf[3]	1910–76	1948–73	Westpoint, MS	Post-war Chicago	Smokestack Lightning	vcl + hca + gtr (with band)
'Big' Joe Turner	1911–85	1938–80s	Kansas City, MO	Jazz/Jump	Roll 'em Pete	vcl (with band)
Robert Johnson	1911–38	1936–37	Hazlehurst, MS	Mississippi	Crossroad Blues	vcl + ac gtr
Sam 'Lightnin'' Hopkins	1912–82	1959–70s (?)	Centerville, TX	Country	Mojo Hand	vcl + gtr
Muddy Waters[4]	1915–83	1941–42; 1948–80s	Rolling Fork, MS	Post-war Chicago	Hoochie Coochie Man	vcl + el gtr (with band)
Memphis Slim[5]	1915–88	1940–81	Memphis, TN	Urban	Every Day I Have the Blues	vcl + pno (with band)
John Lee Hooker	1917–2001	1948–90s	Clarksdale, MS	Idiosyncratic	Boogie Chillen	vcl + el gtr + foot tapping
Professor Longhair[6]	1918–80	1949–80	Bogalusa, LA	New Orleans	Bald Head; Big Chief	vcl + pno (with band)

(continued)

Name	Born–Died	Recording	Birth place	Style	Example	Instruments
'BB' King[7]	1925–	1949–now	Indianola, MS	Urban	Sweet Sixteen	vcl + el gtr (with band)
'Little' Walter Jacobs	1930–68	1947–67	Marksville, LA	Post-war Chicago	My Babe	vcl + hca (with band)
'Buddy' Guy	1936–	1958–now	Lettsworth, LA	Chicago	First Time I Met the Blues	vcl + gtr (with band)

Abbreviations

States: Arkansas (AR); Georgia (GA); Louisiana (LA); Mississippi (MS); Missouri (MO); Tennessee (TN); Texas (TX).

Instruments: acoustic (ac); electric (el); guitar (gtr); harmonica (hca); piano (pno); saxophone (sax); vocal (singing) (vcl).

Footnotes

1. Hudson Woodbridge/Whittaker (he grew up in Tampa, Florida)
2. Major Merriweather
3. Chester Burnett
4. McKinley Morganfield
5. John Len; recorded as Peter Chatman
6. Henry Byrd
7. Riley B King

BOX 13.3 Themes in blues music

Themes usually absent from blues lyrics
- Disadvantage
  - –racism from whites
  - –lynching
  - –slavery, serfdom/sharecropping system
  - –segregation
  - –worse pay and working conditions
  - –disenfranchisement
- Commentary on war
- Commentary on political systems
- Commentary on gender inequalities
- Commentary on lifestyles

Themes commonly present in blues lyrics
- Feelings
- Sex and sexual relationships: sex, bliss, violence, desertion, jealousy
- Having a good time
- Money: poverty, employment, consumerism
- Misfortunes and circumstances
- Crime and penal system
- Disease and death
- Migration
- Substance (ab)use

What is absent from blues lyrics

The focus of blues songs is predominantly personal rather than social or political. Whilst they may express misery or rail against it, they are not primarily 'protest' songs criticising leaders, such as Bob Dylan's 'With God on Our Side',[23] or commenting on social mores, as in the work of the African-American nationalist group, The Last Poets.[24] One can speculate that people need a certain freedom from oppression and disadvantage to be able to produce and listen to such lyrics.

Blues lyrics do include reference to events and situations as they impact on the individual. Natural disasters are well attested, particularly floods and the boll weevil infestation of cotton crops. 'Sales Tax' by the Mississippi Sheiks recorded just that – the impact of an increase in prices due to a new tax.[25] Many songs refer to armed service in various wars – World War II, Korea, Vietnam and Iraq. The financial Great Depression provides a backdrop to songs of that era – 'Nobody Knows You When You're Down and Out' paints a picture of financial ruin but as a personal narrative, not a macroeconomic phenomenon.[26]

The general absence of socio-political commentary illustrates some of the differences between oral and literary tradition. Lynching is not a part of the collective vocabulary, but is captured in the literary, crafted song 'Strange Fruit'.[27] Work songs refer to being chased by the 'sergeant': Jimmy Reed writes in a more literary way about the 'Big Boss Man'.[28]

Racism from whites is not normally attested, but there are references to colour shades (and associated characteristics) within the African-American range of skin tones – yellow, red, brown and black, with black sometimes seen negatively in relation to the others.

What is present in blues lyrics

Emotions, both positive and negative, are frequently featured. These are often set in a narrative context of antecedent, perceived cause and of consequences including coping or action. Negative emotion – the blues – is often given an additional title denoting its putative cause: empty bed blues, lonesome blues, down-and-out blues and the long-way-from-home blues. These feelings are regarded as natural and understandable, not pathological, even when very intense.

The antecedent causes of these feelings relate to common social circumstances – relationships, money/employment, sickness – and to more detailed causal explanations including superstition and black magic.

Many blues songs are about courtship, sexual relationships and sexual gratification. This seems a permitted topic, which may be related to the context of music performance, in particular dances for couples. The degree of sexual explicitness, both directly and through allegorical images, contrasts with the prudishness of contemporaneous US (white) cinema. Prostitution is often casually mentioned as a fact of life. Apart from a pragmatic approach to sexual gratification, blues lyrics refer to many aspects of sexual relationships: teenage bliss (often most apparent in more commercial recordings); loneliness, separation and loss; jealousy. Domestic violence is occasionally referred to, as are violent thoughts[29] and actual murder, including women killing their partners.[30,31]

Another common theme, related to the performance context, is partying, dancing, music, clubs, and generally having a good time.

Money issues are frequently covered either as a primary subject or as backdrop. Lack of money is intimately linked to unemployment. Presence of money is celebrated through consumerism – often a car; sometimes jewellery is mentioned.

Reference to crime and the penal system is normal in prison work songs, but it crops up in blues, often linked to violent thoughts and actions. Non-violent crime is rarely referred to although robbery has been the subject of at least one song.[32]

Disease and death both feature as recorded misfortunes reasonably often. Of individual diseases, tuberculosis is commonly mentioned.[33,34] Dying is sometimes referred to, more often it is the news of the death of a loved one.[35,36]

There is little reference to mental illness. John Lee Hooker's 'Going Mad' and 'Madman' are references to intense love.[37,38] There is equally little reference to healthcare and consultations. Oden sings in 'Goin' Down Slow':

> don't send no doctor – doctor can't do no good,
> it's my fault – never done the things I should.[39]

Smith refers to spa treatment in 'Hot Springs Blues', which seems improbably luxurious.[40]

There were two issues that could appear as *either* a cause *or* a result of the blues – travel and substance abuse.

Migration was very common and, like the Promised Land for Old Testament Jews, stood as a symbol for emancipation – employment at better rates, greater economic independence, and freedom from the monopolistic serfdom of the sharecropper system. Nevertheless it involved uprooting from local communities and their social support, as well as a harsher climate. 'Going back down South – where the weather suits my clothes', sings Buddy Guy, himself originally from Louisiana.[41] Many musicians had a touring lifestyle. The ability to get free long-distance transport by illegally riding freight trains allowed some people to move around as 'hobos'. The structures of the US as a federation of states with different laws encouraged people in trouble to move to a different jurisdiction.

Dealing with emotional problems through substance abuse – and the problems this can cause – is a common theme. Niles quotes an early blues song in which morphine is used to commit suicide.[42] The blues era saw wide variations in drugs of choice and in legality. In 1900, morphine could be bought over the counter and cocaine was a key constituent of Coca-Cola®. By 1920 there was prohibition and a violent swing against intoxicants (narcotics). This facilitated profitable illegal operations, which continue to this day. Alcohol has been the main drug of choice in the US for blacks and whites, and numerous lyrics refer to it. Cannabis is infrequently referred to, as are harder drugs including opiates and cocaine.

One can compare the themes of blues songs with the complaints of people who come to hospital after taking an overdose in the UK. People who have taken overdoses are often relatively powerless and socially deprived, but they do not complain of inability to vote, a Labour government, capitalism, or a high unemployment rate. They do complain of personal adversity (e.g. loss of job, loss of partner, debt, money worries, health worries) and the emotional consequences of such issues. Even in patients who had been admitted to hospital, 89% identified this kind of problem as the reason for first contact with mental health services as opposed to 11% giving mental illness as a reason.[43]

THEORETICAL BACKGROUND
Functions and effects of music

I argue that there are physical and mental benefits to music – for the musician and for the audience, and through the interaction between them, particularly in a participatory oral tradition, and particularly if singing, dancing, and clapping are involved, as would often be the case.

It is important to acknowledge the many overlaps involved. There are historic interconnections between music, poetry, dance, song, chant, ritual (usually spiritual), memory, group cohesion,[44] rites of passage and states of altered consciousness.[45] Contemporary models of physics imply that vibration, and therefore rhythm, is an inherent aspect of matter at a sub-atomic level; at a macroscopic level, the human body and life-cycle have many rhythms.[46] According to Babatunde Olatunji, 'Rhythm is the soul of life because the whole universe revolves around rhythm, and when we get out of rhythm, that's when we get into trouble'.[47]

These interconnecting elements can be divided into intrapersonal relationships within ourselves, to interpersonal relationships between people, and to transpersonal relationships involving transcendence and immanence. I will review potential benefits by dividing them into intrapersonal and interpersonal/transpersonal.

Intrapersonal benefits

Music provides a sense of personal competence/mastery/agency.[48] The detailed qualitative study of DeNora reports that choosing specific music to listen to constitutes a personal narrative ('discourse of self'), with access to recall of significant past experiences and their digestion ('composting'), control and self-regulation of current feelings, and the power to thereby generate one's future identity.[49] Music can provide a space–time which allows retreat, reordering, and refreshment – *reculer pour mieux sauter* (stepping back in order to jump better),[50] or a 'virtual reality' in which 'one registers oneself to oneself as an object of self-knowledge'.[51] Music is seen as a way of attaining intrapersonal attunement which is linked to meditation, ecstasy, and spiritual experiences.[52]

Music clearly affects the subjective mood of normal individuals, and is regarded as a potent technique for the experimental manipulation of moods.[53,54] Rhythmic sounds, both musical and non-musical, are recommended for self-soothing by the Dialectical Behaviour Therapy self-help website.[55]

One of the features of music in general, and blues in particular, is its rhythmicity. This can be reflected in the movement of performers and audience. A subset of this concerns breathing and singing. Singing involves controlling the breath and usually, breathing using the diaphragm, as well as intercostal muscles. This type of breathing is advocated in relaxation exercises. There are reasons to believe that rhythmic activity, particularly if bilateral, is beneficial to health. Because muscles contain receptors, movement links sensory and motor parts of the brain and helps people attune to their bodies. This is also referred to as 'embodiment', which is often considered to be important for mental and physical health. There is a long history in Judaic and Christian traditions of splitting the current material world and associated bodily pleasures from mental and spiritual activity and rewards hereafter. Such a split is not necessarily healthy and could be linked to obscure disorders including somatisation and coenestopathic states.[56] Psychological trauma may alienate people's minds from their bodies.[57] Husserl described movement as 'the mother of all cognition'.[58]

Interpersonal and transpersonal benefits

Song and rhythm may remind us of the soothing effects of cooing and rocking when babies (rocking has to be at least 60 cycles per minute, equivalent to all but the slowest tempo).[59] Mothers/care-givers have a distinctive singing style for infants which has an interpersonal, emotion-regulating effect on the baby, and interchanges which are apparently verbal have musical qualities and soothing effects.[60,61] Music and rhythm can modify various physiological measures including EEG, heart rate, breathing rate and oxygen utilisation.[62]

Sacks has written of the communal and spiritual values of rhythm, chanting and dance.[63] In a similar sense, Kossak refers to interpersonal attunement – the synchrony and complementarity between individuals, including play, attachment and the therapeutic relationship.[64]

A number of religious practices involve breathing exercises (as does non-religious meditation), and others involve repetitive recitation, chanting or incantation (indeed, Qur'an means recitation), all of which have similar effects to singing.

The analysis of lyrical content shows that blues involves expression of emotions. It is important to point out that this is in an open, culturally normal, and acceptable way – in contrast to the secretive shame associated with psychiatric problems in the UK, or even the luxurious private experience of American psychoanalysis. Singing the blues could be regarded as a non-stigmatising, reparative ceremony akin to that described by Warner.[65] Art therapists traditionally emphasise the importance of 'witnessing', which suggests the added value of singing/performing in front of an audience.[66]

Although having the blues is not seen as pathological, having a concurrent mental disorder does not seem to be an obstacle to musicianship in the related area of jazz, and surprisingly little hindrance to musical appreciation.[67,68] In fact, music is reported to reduce negative symptoms of schizophrenia.[69]

Blues music is often dance music and dance embodies emotional expression; it is also a feature of some religious practices (most famously the Sufi 'Whirling Dervishes'). Dance provides a physical activity that promotes both physical and mental health. Dance, physically and emotionally, connects the individual with a partner or participants, and also connects the dancer as audience to the musician-performer. Kreutz investigated Dutch and German tango dancers; although this is obviously a different social context from dancing to blues, the literature and results appear relevant, with dancing seen as mood-improving, involving self-expression, and a way of maintaining and developing social contact.[70]

Research shows considerable congruence between community arts projects, the principles of 'recovery' in mental health, and some common psychological functions of music (*see* Table 13.3).[71]

TABLE 13.3 Comparison of community arts, 'recovery' and music functions

Advantages of community arts[72]	Recovery principles[73]	Music functions[74]
Pleasure	Satisfaction	Enjoyment
Achievement	Autonomy/Activity	Agency
Skill		

(*continued*)

Advantages of community arts[72]	Recovery principles[73]	Music functions[74]
Meaning	Meaning/Purpose/Role	
Cooperation/less social isolation	Social connection	Relationships
Respect	Respect	
More tolerance	Reduced stigma	
Pride in local traditions and culture	Identity	Identity
Increased employment	Income	
	Hope	
	Accommodation	

Neuropsychology

Humans are characterised by their excessive development of the cerebral neocortex – in two halves. This chapter is written in words, we talk in words and analyse in words – which relates to only 50% of our neocortex. In very oversimplified terms, for most people, the right, so-called 'non-dominant' hemisphere is a silent partner; in fact, it deals with emotional material and responds in a holistic rather than analytic and sequential way. The left hemisphere deals predominantly with verbal material, that is words and mathematical symbols (verbal has come to mean oral as opposed to written – I use it here in its earlier meaning of related to words). The right hemisphere deals mainly with appreciation and expression of emotions, music and other non-verbal material (including speech prosody).[75] It is an irony of psychiatry and 'talking treatments' that we spend so much time and effort using left hemisphere tactics (words and sequential analysis) to deal with right hemisphere problems (emotions and holistic apprehensions). The potential of music is to cross the divide and join the two half-spheres, as song involves both words and music.

Mirroring the doctor-patient (therapist-client) interaction

The interaction between doctor and patient – or therapist and client – occurs within certain boundaries and blues music mirrors this in certain ways. Box 13.4 outlines some obvious shared characteristics. A consultation arises in a context – the participants have their histories and experience. There is an overt or ostensible purpose. There is a structure or process and rules governing dialogue. There is an agreed language. Certain subjects are permitted, while others are off-limits and usually unspoken. Irrespective of the overt, primary purpose, a social interaction takes place that will convey much information about the social status of each participant and their relationship to each other. Moreover, creativity and interactive play can be valid, if not essential, components of psychotherapy.[76] Similar components apply to the interaction between musicians and audience.

BOX 13.4 Similarities between a medical consultation and the blues

- Social context
- Overt/primary purpose
- Structure – beginning, middle, end
- Rules of engagement – who speaks when
- Practicalities – language
- Context – what is (not) spoken
- Social markers – pragmatics, vocabulary
- Interactions – difference, antagonism, bonding

Doctors are trained to ask certain questions (*see* Box 13.5), although in practice this varies enormously according to speciality, context and individual practitioner. Much of this is to establish background as a baseline for change, as well as probing for current symptoms. The process is called 'history-taking' – it can feel as though something is being taken from the patient, transformed into a diagnosis, and handed back (or even retained – purloined); a process which can be experienced as positive or negative.[77]

BOX 13.5 Structure of the medical enquiry

What's wrong?	Presenting complaint
Background to what's wrong	History of complaint
What's been wrong before?	Past medical and surgical history
	Past psychiatric history
Current treatment	Medication history
Genetic background (illnesses in relatives)	Family history
Personal background/biography	Personal history
Current circumstances	Social history
Normal mental state	Premorbid personality
Standard questions	Review of systems or mental state examination

CONCLUSION

In summary, blues music represents a relatively recent cultural expression originating in migration and admixture. It is strongly rhythmic and often linked to audience participation and dance. Having the blues is not seen as a pathological, socially excluding state but as a normal emotion. Expressing the blues musically, listening to it, and dancing to it, has mental health benefits. There are a number of similarities between listening to the blues and listening to a patient; in either case, understanding the origins and context, and the process of attunement makes the experience more rewarding.

APPLICATION TO TEACHING

Writing a chapter in a book is a very different exercise to running a workshop or other teaching session. In teaching, I use the music as a practical illustration of listening skills and in a group context it is valuable to elicit and reflect on a range of responses to the same recording. Attending to what is said (and not said) as well as how it is said has lessons for a clinical context. Participants may have a range of exposure to blues music and also a range of acquired opinions or prejudices. I have a particular interest in the oral tradition, and this can be illustrated in many ways. There are a number of formulaic verses that crop up in many different songs. There are recordings that illustrate interaction between musician and audience,[78] preacher and congregation,[79] leader and chorus,[80] as well as more complex interactions.[81] I also consider that hemispheric lateralisation is largely ignored in mental health work. Some practitioners will be particularly interested in the use of music and rhythm for self-soothing. Finally, many 'recovery' principles are evident in the blues story, most centrally those of self-expression, finding meaning, and the overlap with spirituality. As Holiday says, 'blues to me is like being very sad, very sick, going to church, being very happy'.[82] Many of these points could equally be conveyed by other cross-over or hybrid music, such as hip hop, reggae or bhangra.

The experience of a journey, in which we lose at least some of our heritage and support and are exposed to new experience, is at the foundation of the blues and of great relevance to an increasingly globalised and changing world. It is also an archetypal allegory of personal development, which has been retold over the centuries, including in influential texts 'The Epic of Gilgamesh', Homer's *Odyssey* and Dante's *Divine Comedy*. To illustrate, Dante starts 'in the middle of the journey'; one of Robert Johnson's most haunting recordings is 'Crossroads Blues'. 'The Yoruba have the idea of the crossroads, the point where the spirit world and this world intersect. Certain things attract the spirits to a crossroads. One is music, another is stories. The spirits love to listen to both'.[83]

ACKNOWLEDGEMENTS

I am grateful to my wife, Fiona Russell Dodwell, for many fruitful discussions and advice.

BIBLIOGRAPHY

Charters S. *The Bluesmen*. New York, NY: Oak Publications; 1967.

Davis F. *The History of the Blues*. London: Martin & Warburg Ltd; 1995.

Lomax A. *The Land Where the Blues Began*. London: Minerva; 1994.

Oliver P. *The Story of the Blues*. Harmondsworth, Middlesex: Penguin; 1972.

Oliver P. *Blues Fell this Morning: meaning in the blues*. 2nd ed. Cambridge: Cambridge University Press; 1990.

REFERENCES

1 Hartshorne, cited in Storr A. *Music and the Mind*. London: HarperCollins Publishers; 1993. p. 4.

2 Davis F. *The History of the Blues*. London: Martin & Warburg Ltd; 1997. p. 57.

3 Holiday B. Spoken introduction to 'Fine and Mellow' (B Holiday). *Billie Holiday: The Real Lady Sings the Blues*. London: Boulevard Records; Boulevard 4113 (Vinyl); reissued 1973. Side 1, Track 4.

4 Skrabanek P, McCormick J. *Follies and Fallacies in Medicine*. Glasgow: Tarragon Press; 1989. p. 79.

5 Carmack HJ, Bates BR, Harter LM. Narrative constructions of health care issues and policies: the case of President Clinton's apology-by-proxy for the Tuskegee syphilis experiment. *JMH*. 2008; **29**: 89–109.

6 Hart M, Stevens J, Lieberman F. *Drumming at the Edge of Magic: a journey into the spirit of percussion*. New York, NY: HarperCollins Publishers; 1990. p. 224.

7 Jackson B (editor). *Wake Up Dead Man: Black convict work songs from Texas prisons*. Somerville, MA: Rounder Records; 2013 (Vinyl); Library of Congress #74–750921; 1975.

8 Davis A, Gardner BB, Gardner MR. *Deep South: a social anthropological study of caste and class*. Chicago, IL: University of Chicago Press; 1941. pp. 276–99.

9 Swinton P. Mississippi Sheiks [CD booklet]. *Mississippi Sheiks: Show Me What You Got*. Guildford, Surrey: Catfish Records; Catfish KACD124 (CD); 1999.

10 Jackson B (editor). *Wake Up Dead Man: Black convict work songs from Texas prisons*. Somerville, MA: Rounder Records; 2013 (Vinyl); Library of Congress #74–750921; 1975.

11 Lomax A. Liner notes. *Southern Journey*. Volume 13: Earliest Times: Georgia Sea Islands songs for everyday living. Cambridge, MA: Rounder Records; Rounder CD 1713 (CD); 1998.

12 Gates JM and Congregation. *You Mother Heartbreakers* (1929). In: Charters SB (compiler and editor). *An Introduction to Gospel Singing*. New York, NY: RBF Records; RF-5 (Vinyl); 1962. Side 1,Track 4.

13 Charters S. *The Bluesmen*. New York, NY: Oak Publications; 1967. p. 15.

14 Lorca FG. 1960. 'Theory and Function of the Duende'. (Translated from 'Juego y teoria del duende', lecture first given 1933.) In: Gili JL (selector and translator). *Lorca*. Harmondsworth, Middlesex: Penguin; 1960. pp. 127–39.

15 Harrison JL. *Themis: a study of the social origins of Greek religion*. London: Merlin Press; 1963.

16 Lomax A. Liner notes. *Southern Journey*. Volume 13: Earliest Times: Georgia Sea Islands songs for everyday living. Cambridge, MA: Rounder Records; Rounder 1713 (CD); 1998.

17 Dodwell D. Kalevala or Keats: poetic traditions as a model for multidisciplinary miscommunication and team splitting. *J Psychiatr Ment Health Nurs*. 2008; **15**(7): 547–51.

18 Holiday B. Spoken introduction to 'Fine and Mellow' (1939). *Billie Holiday: The Real Lady Sings the Blues*. B Holiday. London: Boulevard Records; Boulevard 4113 (Vinyl); reissued 1973. Side 1, Track 4.

9 Larkin C (editor). *The Guinness Who's Who of Blues*. Enfield, Middlesex: Guinness Publishing; 1993.

20 Morganfield M [Muddy Waters]. 'I Feel Like Going Home' (1947). *Back in the Early Days: Volumes 1 and 2*. Muddy Waters. Norfolk, England: Syndicate Chapter Records; SC001/2 (Vinyl two-record set); reissued 1971. Volume 1, Side 1, Track 1.

21 Morganfield M [Muddy Waters]. 'Where's My Woman Been?' (1949). *Muddy Waters Rare & Unissued*. Universal City, CA: Chess Masters; CXMP2057 (Vinyl); reissued 1985. Side 1, Track 7.

22 Morganfield M [Muddy Waters]. 'Country Boy' (1951). *Back in the Early Days: Volumes 1 & 2*. Muddy Waters. Norfolk, England: Syndicate Chapter Records; SC001/2 (Vinyl two-record set); reissued 1971. Volume 1, Side 1, Track 7.

23 Dylan R. 'With God on Our Side'. New York, NY: Special Rider Music; 1963.

24 The Last Poets. 'Jones Comin' Down'. *Beats Rhyme + Revolution: the best of the Last Poets 1970–1985*. Watford, Herts: Music Collection International; MCCD 311 (CD); 1997. Track 2.

25 Mississippi Sheiks. 'Sales Tax' (1934). *Mississippi Sheiks: Show Me What You Got*. Guildford, Surrey: Catfish Records; KATCD124 (CD); reissued 1999. Track 12.

26 Smith B. 'Nobody Knows You When You're Down and Out'. Words and music by J. Cox (Colombia 144451-D; 1929). *Any Woman's Blues*. London: CBS Records; CBS66262 (Vinyl two-record set); reissued 1970. Side 3, Track 5.

27 Holiday B. 1939. 'Strange Fruit'. Words by L. Allan (A. Meeropol) (1935). New York, NY: Commodore Records; 526 (Vinyl); 1939. Track 1, 78 rpm.

28 Reed J. 'Big Boss Man' (1960). *The Best of Jimmy Reed*. Hollywood, CA: GNP Crescendo Records; GNPS/2–10006 (Vinyl two-record set); reissued 1974. Side 3, Track 3.

29 Johnson R. '32–20 Blues' (1936). Originally issued as Vocalion 03445. *Robert Johnson: King of the Delta Blues Singers*. London: CBS Records; CBS 62456 (Vinyl); reissued 1966. Side 1, Track 6.

30 Smith B. 'Send Me to the 'lectric Chair' (1927). Composed by G. Brooks. *Bessie Smith: The Empress*. London: CBS Records; CBS66264 (Vinyl two-record set); reissued 1971. Side 3, Track 5.

31 Fitzgerald E, Jordan L. 'Stone Cold Dead in the Market (He Had it Coming)' (1946). *1946: The R&B Hits* (Various Artists). London: Indigo Records; IGOCD 2060 (CD); reissued 1997. Track 12.

32 Kenner C. 'They Took My Money' (1964). *New Orleans R&B: Volume 2*. Bexhill-on-Sea, Sussex: Flyright Records; LP4709 (Vinyl); re-released 1974. Side 2, Track 5.

33 Spivey V. 'TB Blues' (1927). Original 78 OKEH8494. *Ma Rainey & The Classic Blues Singers*. London: CBS Records; CBS52798 (Vinyl): reissued 1970. Side 2, Track 7.

34 Hooker JL. 'No Friend Around' (1950). Original recording B8010. *John Lee Hooker . . . No Friend Around*. Diss, Norfolk: Red Lightnin' Records; RL003 (Vinyl); re-released 1970. Side 1, Track 7.

35 Oden J (St Louis Jimmy). 'Goin' Down Slow'. Originally released as Bluebird B8889B (Vinyl); 1941. 78 rpm.

36 House S. 'Death Letter Blues' (1965). Original recording reissued. *Son House: The Original Delta Blues*. Los Angeles, CA: Columbia; COL489891 2 (CD); 1998. Track 1.

37   Hooker JL. 'Goin' Mad Blues' (1948). Original recording D1104. *John Lee Hooker: The Classic Early Years 1948–1951*. London: JSP Records; JSPLD 7703A (4-CD set); reissued 2002. Disc A, Track 12.

38   Hooker JL. 'Mad Man Blues' (1950). Original recording D1104. *John Lee Hooker: The Classic Early Years 1948–1951*. London: JSP Records; JSPLD 7703C (4-CD set); reissued 2002. Disc C, Track 21.

39   Oden J (St Louis Jimmy). 'Goin' Down Slow'. Originally released as Bluebird B8889B (Vinyl); 1941. 78 rpm.

40   Smith B. 'Hot Springs Blues' (1927). Words by B Smith. *Bessie Smith: The Empress*. London: CBS Records; CBS66264 (Vinyl 2-record set); reissued 1971. Side 3, Track 6.

41   Guy B. 'Stone Crazy' (1961). Original released by Chess. *In the Beginning*. Diss, Norfolk: Red Lightnin' Records; RL001 (Vinyl); undated. Side 2, Track 2.

42   Niles A. Introduction. In: Handy WC (editor). *Blues: an anthology*. New York, NY: Albert & Charles Boni; 1926. Bedford, MA: Applewood Books; undated reprint. pp 1–24.

43   Rogers A, Pilgrim D, Lacey R. *Experiencing Psychiatry: users' views of services*. Houndmills, Basingstoke: Macmillan; 1993.

44   Storr A. *Music and the Mind*. London: HarperCollins Publishers; 1993. pp. 16–17.

45   Hart M, Stevens J, Lieberman F. *Drumming at the Edge of Magic: a journey into the spirit of percussion*. New York, NY: HarperCollins Publishers; 1990. pp. 161–77.

46   Ibid. pp. 118–23.

47   Ibid. p. 212.

48   Storr, op. cit. pp. 101–5; DeNora T. Music as a technology of the self. *Poetics*. 1999; **27**: 31–56.

49   DeNora op. cit.

50   Storr, op. cit. p. 105

51   DeNora, op. cit.

52   Kossak MS. Therapeutic attachment: a transpersonal view of expressive arts therapy. *Art Psychother*. 2009; **36**(1): 13–18.

53   Smith JL, Noon J. Objective measurement of mood change induced by contemporary music. *J Psychiatr Ment Health Nurs*. 1998; **5**: 403–8.

54   Thaut MH, de l'Etoile SK. The effects of music on mood state-dependent recall. *J Music Ther*. 1993; **30**(2): 70–80.

55   DBT Self Help website. Self-soothe. Available at: www.dbtselfhelp.com/html/print053.html (accessed 17 May 2010).

56   Dupré E. Les Cénestopathies. *Mouvement Médical*. 1913; 3–22. Translated by M Rohde as 'Coenestopathic states'. In: Hirsch SR, Shepherd M (editors). *Themes and Variations in European Psychiatry*. Bristol: John Wright & Sons; 1974. pp. 385–94.

57   Totton N. Foreign bodies: recovering the history of body psychotherapy. In: Staunton T (editor). *Body Psychotherapy*. Hove: Brunner-Routledge; 2002. pp. 7–26.

58   Husserl cited in Gibbs RW. *Embodiment and Cognitive Science*. New York, NY: Cambridge University Press; 2006. p. 28.

59   Bowlby J. *Attachment and Loss. Volume 1: Attachment*. 2nd ed. London: Penguin Books; 1984. pp. 291–6.

60   Peretz I. Listen to the brain: a biological perspective on musical emotions. In: Juslin

PN, Sloboda JA (editors). *Music and Emotion.* Oxford: Oxford University Press; 2001. pp. 105–34.

61 Storr A. *Music and the Mind.* London: HarperCollins Publishers; 1993. pp 8–9.

62 Moerman D. *Meaning, Medicine and the 'Placebo Effect'.* Cambridge: Cambridge University Press; 2002. p. 143.

63 Sacks O. *Musicophilia: tales of music on the brain.* London: Picador; 2008. pp. 266–9.

64 Kossak MS. Therapeutic attachment: a transpersonal view of expressive arts therapy. *Art Psychother.* 2009; 36(1): 13–18.

65 Warner R. *Recovery from Schizophrenia: psychiatry and political economy.* 3rd ed. Hove: Brunner-Routledge; 2004. p. 179.

66 Jones P. *The Arts Therapies: a revolution in healthcare.* Hove: Brunner-Routledge; 2005. pp. 262–6.

67 Wills GI. Forty lives in the bebop business: mental health in a group of eminent jazz musicians. *Br J Psychiatr.* 2003; 183: 225–59.

68 Sacks O. *Musicophilia: tales of music on the brain.* London: Picador; 2008. p. 331.

69 Edwards J. Music therapy in the treatment and management of mental disorders. *Ir J Psychol Med.* 2006; 23(1): 33–5; Gold C, Heldal TO, Dahle T, Wigram T. Music therapy for schizophrenia or schizophrenia-like illnesses. *Cochrane Database of Systematic Reviews.* 2005, Issue 2.

70 Kreutz G. Does partnered dance promote health? The case of Tango Argentino. *JRSH.* 2008; 128(2): 79–84.

71 Matarasso F. *Use or Ornament? The Social Impact of Participation in the Arts.* Stroud, Gloucestershire: Comedia; 1997.

72 Ibid.

73 Department of Health. *The Journey to Recovery: the Government's vision for mental health care.* London: Department of Health Publications; 2001; Shepherd G, Boardman J, Slade M. *Making Recovery a Reality.* London: Sainsbury Centre for Mental Health; 2008.

74 Laiho S. The psychological functions of music in adolescence. *Nord J Music Ther.* 2004; 13(1): 47–63.

75 Springer SP, Deutsch G. *Left Brain, Right Brain.* 3rd ed. New York, NY: WH Freeman & Co; 1989; Cutting J. *The Right Hemisphere and Psychiatric Disorders.* Oxford: Oxford University Press; 1990; Juslin PN. Communicating emotion in music performance: a review and theoretical framework. In: Juslin PN, Sloboda JA (editors). *Music and Emotion.* Oxford: Oxford University Press; 2001. pp. 305–7; Mula M, Trimble MR. Music and madness, neuropsychiatric aspects of music. *Clin Med.* 2009; 9(1): 83–6.

76 Winnicott DW. *Playing and Reality.* Harmondsworth, Middlesex: Penguin Books; 1985. pp. 62–3.

77 Rogers A, Pilgrim D, Lacey R. *Experiencing Psychiatry: users' views of services.* Houndmills, Basingstoke: Macmillan; 1993.

78 King BB. 'Nightlife'. *Blues is King.* Hayes, Middlesex: EMI Records/His Master's Voice; HMVCSD 3608 (Vinyl); 1967. Side 1, Track 4.

79 Gates JM and Congregation. *You Mother Heartbreakers* (1929). In: Charters SB (compiler and editor). *An Introduction to Gospel Singing.* New York, NY: RBF Records; RF-5 (Vinyl); 1962.

80 Jackson J & Group. 'I'm in The Bottom' (1965). *Wake Up Dead Man: Black convict work songs from Texas prisons.* Somerville, MA: Rounder Records; 2013 (Vinyl): 1975. Side 1, Track 4.

81 Veasley E, Phillips M, Mitchell T. 'Captain Don't Feel Sorry for a Long Time Man' (1965). *Wake Up Dead Man: Black convict work songs from Texas prisons.* Somerville, MA: Rounder Records; 2013 (Vinyl): 1975. Side 1, Track 5.

82 Holiday B. Spoken introduction to 'Fine and Mellow' (1939). *Billie Holiday: The Real Lady Sings the Blues.* B Holiday. London: Boulevard Records; Boulevard 4113 (Vinyl); reissued 1973. Side 1, Track 4.

83 Hart M, Stevens J, Lieberman F. *Drumming at the Edge of Magic: a journey into the spirit of percussion.* New York, NY: HarperCollins Publishers; 1990. pp. 242.

Index